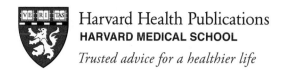

## Harvard Health Publications
### HARVARD MEDICAL SCHOOL

*Trusted advice for a healthier life*

Dear Reader,

You've been making health decisions all your life. You probably make the everyday choices—what to eat, when to exercise, and how long to sleep—almost instinctively. You've also encountered occasional medical decisions, like which screening tests to have, which pills to take to prevent illness, or which procedures to undergo to feel better.

At midlife, however, medical decisions are changing and coming more frequently—when to have mammograms, colonoscopies, or bone density tests, for example. You may be trying to decide whether to have bunion surgery or a knee replacement. Or you may be puzzling over the best way to manage your arthritis or irritable bowel syndrome. You know these decisions are important. They can mean identifying and treating a disease while a cure is still possible, or minimizing troublesome symptoms, reducing pain, and preserving mobility.

Yet the lifestyle choices you make can also have an enormous impact on your overall health. Women's health studies have shown that it's never too late to feel better by living better. For example, following a plant-based eating plan may reduce your risks for a number of problems, including heart attack, stroke, diabetes, and Alzheimer's disease. Women who exercise regularly are less likely to feel depressed and anxious and less likely to develop a host of chronic debilitating conditions. And did you know that getting sufficient sleep—from seven to nine hours a night—will not only boost your energy, but also help you lose weight and keep it off?

One thing that always strikes me in dealing with my patients is that women are not just different from men physiologically and emotionally, but different from one another as well—in their genetic endowment as much as their life experiences. And each woman ages differently, too. As a result, your individual health concerns aren't likely to be the same as they were 30 years ago, nor are they likely to be identical to those of your friends.

This report is about health, not disease. Its goal is not to serve as an exhaustive compendium of treatments, but rather to help you determine the conditions for which you are at greatest risk and do your best to avoid them. It will also help you better manage chronic conditions that may erode your quality of life and develop strategies for maintaining an active, productive life going forward. It is designed to give you the information to make choices today that will ensure you the best health possible tomorrow.

Sincerely

Hope Ricciotti, M.D.
*Medical Editor*

# Taking stock of your health at midlife

Midlife can be a woman's halftime celebration. Not only is it an opportunity to reflect on and rejoice in the life you've lived, but it is also a good time to plan your strategy for the future.

If you're like most women, menopause is likely to give you a new perspective on life and health. Premenstrual syndrome, menstrual discomforts, and reproductive issues are no longer a concern. Hot flashes and other perimenopausal symptoms are gradually disappearing. As you move into the sixth decade of life, you may be feeling the burst of energy and optimism that anthropologist Margaret Mead famously termed "postmenopausal zest."

In the following decades, your health focus will continue to shift. Initially, you are likely to be most concerned with preventing or managing the conditions that become more prevalent as estrogen declines—for example, osteoporosis, heart disease, sexual dysfunction, skin changes, and bladder control. Once you have reached your eighth or ninth decade, you may be more focused on staying strong enough to live independently, pursue the hobbies that give you pleasure, and enjoy your family and friends.

Every step of the way, the choices you make can have a real impact on your health. So how do you start planning for a healthy future? First, acknowledge what you can't control. Then put your energies into changing what you can change—for the better.

## What you can't control

Even though you can't change the following factors, knowing your risks can help you plan for the future.

**Age.** As people grow older, their bodies undergo gradual physical changes that are normal and inevitable. Such changes begin with random genetic mistakes that occur as cells divide and DNA is improperly copied. Over time the cellular damage accumulates, affecting every tissue and organ of the body. These changes occur at different rates throughout the body and from person to person.

**Family medical history.** If an immediate family member—a parent or sibling—developed a problem such as heart disease or cancer, especially if it occurred early in life, it could mean that you are at risk as well. Shared genes explain some of this risk, but so do shared lifestyles, such as the food you eat and how active you are.

## What you can control

It may surprise you to know that what you can control often affects your health much more than the factors you can't change. For all the media coverage of genetic discoveries, for example, it turns out that many genes are responsive to lifestyle changes such as improvements in diet and exercise. With healthful lifestyle changes, disease-promoting genes become less active, while those that protect you become more active. Here are just a few such factors to consider.

**Whether you smoke.** Roughly one in five American women smokes. If you are one of them, kicking the habit may be the single most important thing you can do to improve your health, simultaneously reducing your risks of heart disease, stroke, and various cancers.

**What you eat.** Consuming a healthy diet on a regular basis is one of the best ways to help prevent—and manage—heart disease, high blood pressure, and type 2 diabetes. Doing so can even reduce your risk of dementia.

**How much you move.** Get active, live longer. Not only that, but live better. Study after study has linked greater amounts of physical activity to improved health.

Intrigued? Turn to the next chapter and start evaluating your own health portfolio, so that you can start making wise investments in your health. ♥

# Understanding your health risks

If you are in midlife or later, you may have already experienced some signs of aging: your joints may ache occasionally, you may not recall names as easily as you once did, and you may not sleep as well as you used to. Many of the chronic conditions that begin to plague women in midlife are due, in part, to declining levels of estrogen, which helps to maintain tissues in the body's reproductive organs as well as in the breasts, brain, bones, bladder, and cardiovascular system. Genetic makeup is also complicit, as are the cumulative effects of normal aging, environmental forces, and lifestyle choices. Death statistics from the CDC illustrate how the leading killers of women change with age (see Table 1, below).

This chapter will give you an idea of the factors likely to put you at greatest risk for a variety of conditions in the years to come. Any measures you can take to protect yourself specifically against a given disease are discussed in each section. Fortunately, many measures reduce risks across the board; the Special Section of this report—"10 steps to a longer and healthier life," beginning on page 20—is devoted to them.

## Table 1: Leading causes of death in women by age, 2013

This chart shows the top 10 causes of death (expressed as a percentage of total deaths) in women at different ages. You can see how the risk of the three leading killers for all ages combined—heart disease, cancer, and chronic lung diseases—changes with age by following the red, yellow, and pink boxes. Chronic lung diseases include asthma and chronic obstructive pulmonary disease (COPD), which itself encompasses two diseases—chronic bronchitis and emphysema. Septicemia refers to blood infections.

| AGE | 45–54 | 55–64 | 65–74 | 75–84 | 85+ |
|-----|-------|-------|-------|-------|-----|
| 1 | Cancer 33% | Cancer 38% | Cancer 36% | Cancer 23% | Heart disease 29% |
| 2 | Heart disease 15% | Heart disease 17% | Heart disease 18% | Heart disease 22% | Cancer 10% |
| 3 | Accidents 10% | Chronic lung diseases 6% | Chronic lung diseases 9% | Chronic lung diseases 8% | Alzheimer's disease 8% |
| 4 | Chronic liver disease 4% | Accidents 4% | Stroke 4% | Stroke 7% | Stroke 7% |
| 5 | Chronic lung diseases 4% | Diabetes 4% | Diabetes 4% | Alzheimer's disease 5% | Chronic lung diseases 5% |
| 6 | Stroke 3% | Stroke 4% | Kidney disease 2% | Diabetes 3% | Influenza and pneumonia 3% |
| 7 | Diabetes 3% | Chronic liver disease 3% | Accidents 2% | Influenza and pneumonia 2% | Accidents 2% |
| 8 | Suicide 3% | Septicemia 2% | Septicemia 2% | Accidents 2% | Diabetes 2% |
| 9 | Septicemia 2% | Kidney disease 2% | Influenza and pneumonia 2% | Kidney disease 2% | Hypertension 2% |
| 10 | Influenza and pneumonia 1% | Influenza and pneumonia 2% | Alzheimer's disease 1.3% | Septicemia 2% | Kidney disease 2% |

RANK

*Source: CDC.*

# Cardiovascular disease

Cardiovascular disease is the leading cause of death in women, killing more women in the United States than all types of cancer combined—290,000 a year for heart disease versus 277,000 for cancer. But heart disease encroaches more stealthily in women than it does in men, with symptoms beginning about a decade later. And it doesn't always manifest itself the same way as it does in men.

As the name implies, cardiovascular disease affects the vessels that wrap around the heart, bringing oxygenated blood to the heart muscle itself. This includes the major coronary arteries, which lie on the surface of the heart, and a web of ever-smaller vessels that branch from the coronary arteries to saturate the heart tissue with blood.

Trouble begins when excess cholesterol—carried through the bloodstream in protein-coated particles known as LDL, or "bad" cholesterol—builds up in artery walls. In a perfect world, you would have sufficient HDL, or "good" cholesterol particles, to sop up the excess and carry it to the liver for disposal. But many women do not have enough HDL. The immune system sees the cholesterol that remains in vessel walls as an invader and launches an inflammatory attack. White blood cells gobble up the cholesterol, becoming engorged with fat and mired in the vessel walls, where many of them die, spilling their contents. In an attempt to isolate the damage, the immune system then encases the area in a fibrous coat, forming atherosclerotic plaque. But because the cholesterol hasn't been eliminated, the inflammatory process persists.

According to the classic model of cardiovascular disease, this plaque can reduce blood flow to the heart, causing chest pain (angina). It can also lead to heart attacks in one of two ways. Plaque can build up inside a coronary artery until it blocks blood flow completely, starving the heart muscle of oxygen and nutrients. Or, more frequently, unstable plaque can rupture under pressure. A blood clot then forms over the ruptured plaque, and it's the clot that blocks the artery.

However, it turns out that there is a third way to develop cardiovascular disease and heart attacks. It involves a condition known as coronary microvascular disease—and while this can affect men, it is more common in women, especially younger women (average age 49).

In microvascular disease, the problem begins not in the major coronary arteries, but in the smaller arteries that branch off those larger vessels. Instead of developing plaques that burrow into the vessel wall or jut into the open passage through which blood flows, the smaller vessels suffer from inflammation that narrows and stiffens them (see Figure 1, below). They can't dilate to increase blood flow in response to the body's demands, so the heart doesn't get all the blood it needs. Moreover, damage to the inner walls of these small vessels can lead to spasms that further reduce blood flow to the heart, causing symptoms such as fatigue, diffuse chest discomfort, shortness of breath, and sometimes heart attacks.

Unfortunately, there are no good tests for detecting microvascular disease, since the standard tests were designed for detecting problems in large vessels. People with symptoms such as chest pain first undergo noninvasive stress tests to determine whether the heart is getting enough blood as oxygen demands increase.

---

## Figure 1: Causes of ischemic heart disease

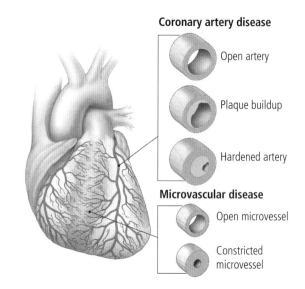

**Coronary artery disease**
- Open artery
- Plaque buildup
- Hardened artery

**Microvascular disease**
- Open microvessel
- Constricted microvessel

Ischemic heart disease is reduced blood flow to the heart. According to the classic model of the disease, trouble begins when plaque builds up inside a coronary artery, which eventually thickens and hardens, obstructing blood flow. The newer view of ischemic heart disease suggests that the tiny vessels feeding the heart can also become stiff and narrow, reducing blood flow.

If these tests indicate reduced blood flow to the heart, the next step is coronary angiography—an x-ray that shows where the vessel is blocked and the size of the obstruction. Once pinpointed, the blockage may be flattened during coronary angioplasty or bypassed with a vessel graft. However, as many as 30% of women with angina have "clear" angiograms. In addition to performing these tests, then, your doctor will place a lot of weight on your family history of heart disease, other medical problems you may have (such as overweight or diabetes) that can contribute to heart disease, and a detailed analysis of your symptoms.

Prevention of microvascular disease involves the same basic measures that you would take to prevent classic heart disease.

## Risk factors

Many factors interact to increase your risk of developing heart disease (see "Calculating your risk," below, to estimate your own risk).

**Age.** After 55, a woman's chance of having a heart attack begins to rise steadily. Not coincidentally, by that time, most women have gone through menopause, and the protective effects of estrogen—raising HDL and lowering LDL cholesterol levels—are disappearing. Postmenopausal women are two to three times as likely to develop heart disease as women the same age who are still menstruating.

**Family history.** You have a strong genetic risk if you have a mother or sister who was diagnosed with

▶ **Heart hint**

Statins are drugs that work by altering the metabolism of cholesterol. They lower "bad" LDL and triglycerides and nudge up "good" HDL. The benefits of statins seem to outweigh the risks (primarily of muscle pain and liver damage) for women with heart disease, but haven't been shown to decrease the risk of a fatal heart attack in healthy women.

However, 2013 guidelines issued by the American College of Cardiology (ACC) and American Heart Association (AHA) recommend considering a statin if your risk of a heart attack or stroke is at least 7.5% in the next decade. If you're at increased risk for heart disease and can't get your LDL cholesterol down to acceptable levels, discuss the matter with your doctor. If you're on the fence, a high-sensitivity test for CRP—an indicator of inflammation—may help you decide.

coronary artery disease before age 65 or a father or brother who developed it before age 55. While your heritage doesn't necessarily consign you to heart disease, it should serve as a signal to be alert for symptoms and to keep other risk factors under control.

**Ethnicity.** African Americans, Mexican Americans, Native Americans, and native Hawaiians are all more likely than people of European descent to develop heart disease. Researchers are still trying to determine how much of the risk stems from genetics and how much from cultural practices.

**Smoking.** Smoking is the leading preventable

## Calculating your risk

Three different calculators are available online to help you estimate your risk of a heart attack in the next 10 years.

**The Framingham Risk Calculator** has been developed and modified over the years based on data from participants in the Framingham Heart Study. You can find it online at http://cvdrisk.nhlbi.nih.gov.

**The Reynolds Risk Score,** based on data from the Women's Health Study, was created to better predict risk in women. It requires the results of a high-sensitivity blood test for C-reactive protein (hsCRP test; see "Inflammation," page 7). The Reynolds calculator is available at www.reynoldsriskscore.org.

**The ACC/AHA Heart Risk Calculator** is based on the 2013 guidelines developed by the American College of Cardiology and the American Heart Association for assessing heart disease risk. Its principal purpose is to help determine whether an individual might benefit from taking a statin. It is at www.cvriskcalculator.com.

The three ask for slightly different information and may yield different results. However, they can give you a general idea of whether you should review your risk factors with your doctor.

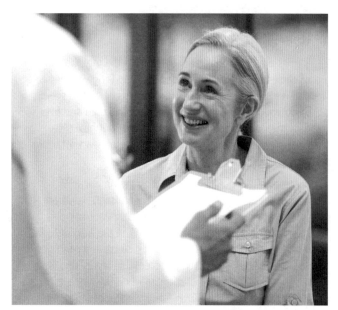

The higher your HDL, or "good" cholesterol, the lower your chances of having a heart attack. Research suggests that every one-point rise in HDL lowers the risk by 2% to 3%.

© Stockbyte | Thinkstock

cause of death in the United States, and one in three smoking-related deaths is from cardiovascular disease. Even nonsmokers increase their heart disease risk by 25% to 30% when they live with smokers. That said, the damage is reversible. Within a year of quitting, former smokers have slashed their risk in half. Fifteen years out, they have erased almost all of it.

**Diabetes.** An adult diagnosed with diabetes has the same high cardiac risk as someone who has already had a heart attack. At least 65% of people with diabetes will die from some type of cardiovascular disease—a death rate that is two to four times that of the general population. Diabetes can also cause chronic kidney disease, which in turn can increase the risk of cardiovascular disease even more. That's because damage to the kidneys' filtering capacity allows substances like renin (which increases blood pressure) to build up in the bloodstream, harming blood vessels.

**Unfavorable cholesterol profile.** The more LDL in your bloodstream, the greater your heart risk. The National Cholesterol Education Program (NCEP), a division of the National Heart, Lung, and Blood Institute of the National Institutes of Health (NIH), has been evaluating the evolving medical evidence on cholesterol for several decades. It categorizes LDL levels below 100 milligrams per deciliter (mg/dL) as opti-

mal, those 100 to 129 as near to above optimal, 130 to 159 as borderline high, 160 to 189 as high, and greater than 190 as very high.

By contrast, the more HDL in your bloodstream, the lower your chances of having a heart attack. Findings from the Framingham Heart Study (a long-running landmark study of factors contributing to heart disease) and elsewhere suggest that every one-point rise in HDL lowers the risk for heart attack 2% to 3%. The NCEP guidelines consider levels of 60 mg/dL or above as protective against heart disease, while levels below 40 mg/dL increase your risk.

**High blood pressure (hypertension).** High blood pressure damages the cells lining arteries, prompting the immune system to mount an inflammatory response that contributes to the development of atherosclerotic plaques. These plaques cause the arteries to stiffen, which drives up blood pressure even more, setting up a vicious circle. If these plaques enlarge, rupture, or break off, they can also lead directly to heart attacks and strokes. The chance of developing complications increases with higher levels of blood pressure.

Your blood pressure reading has two parts. The first and higher number (systolic blood pressure) represents the pressure while the heart is beating and shows how hard the heart works to push blood through the arteries. The second and lower number (diastolic blood pressure), which represents the pressure when the heart is relaxing and refilling with blood between beats, shows how forcefully arteries are being stretched most of the time.

The Joint National Committee on Prevention, Detection, Evaluation, and Treatment of High Blood Pressure defines normal blood pressure as below 120/80 millimeters of mercury (mm Hg), prehypertension as 120–139/80–89, hypertension stage 1 as 140–159/90–99, and hypertension stage 2 as 160/100 or greater. If your systolic and diastolic pressures fall into two different categories—if, for example, your pressure is 130/75—your degree of hypertension will be based on the higher category.

The results of the Systolic Blood Pressure Intervention Trial (SPRINT), reported in November 2015, may change recommendations for treating high blood

## Where's the salt?

To keep your blood pressure in check, it may help to cut back on your salt intake. The 2015–2020 Dietary Guidelines for Americans recommend limiting sodium to 2,300 milligrams (mg) per day for the general population, and suggest that people 51 and older should consume even less—1,500 mg. That's less than half the amount the average American consumes. If you're looking to scale back on salt, you may want to begin with processed foods, which, together with restaurant food, provide most of the sodium in the average person's diet. Following are the top 10 sources of salt, according to the CDC. The ranking is based on both the total sodium content of foods and how often people eat these foods.

1. breads and rolls
2. cold cuts and cured meats
3. pizza
4. poultry (such as breaded chicken strips or nuggets)
5. soups
6. sandwiches
7. cheese
8. pasta dishes (such as spaghetti with meat sauce)
9. meat dishes (such as beef stew or meatloaf with tomato sauce)
10. savory snacks (such as chips and pretzels).

Check the sodium content on the Nutrition Facts panel of every packaged food you buy. It will be listed both in milligrams and as a percentage of the recommended daily sodium allowance per serving.

pressure. That study involved 9,361 people with high blood pressure but not diabetes, 38% of whom were women. Participants were randomly assigned to one of two groups. The first group received conventional blood pressure treatment designed to lower systolic blood pressure to a target of less than 140 mm Hg. The other received more intensive treatment aimed at achieving a lower target—less than 120 mm Hg. The results determined that, over all, participants who were treated intensively had a 25% reduction in risk for heart attacks, strokes, and death from cardiovascular causes, compared with those on conventional therapy. Among participants ages 75 and over, the reduction was 33%. However, women received less benefit than men from the more intensive treatment.

The reduction in cardiovascular events was only 16% for women of all ages, compared with 28% for all men.

Before the SPRINT results came out, doctors had begun to question the wisdom of strict blood pressure goals in older adults. As blood vessels stiffen with age, slightly higher blood pressure values might be needed to keep plenty of blood flowing to the brain and heart, they thought. However, the study results indicate that many older adults may benefit from more intensive therapy. So if you're past age 75 and your systolic blood pressure is over 140 mm Hg, you may want to weigh the potential risks and benefits of lowering it further with your doctor.

In the SPRINT trial, lowering blood pressure to 140 mm Hg or less required an average of two blood pressure medications, and achieving a pressure of 120 mm Hg or less took an average of three drugs. Moreover, the rate of serious adverse effects from therapy, including kidney damage, fainting, and bouts of abnormally low blood pressure, was significantly higher among participants who were more intensively treated.

**Metabolic syndrome.** About 23% of American women have metabolic syndrome, a constellation of attributes that increases the risk of developing diabetes and coronary artery disease. Any woman with three or more of the following meets the diagnostic criteria for metabolic syndrome:

- waist size greater than 35 inches
- blood pressure that is 130/85 mm Hg or higher
- HDL cholesterol that is less than 50 mg/dL
- triglyceride level that is 150 mg/dL or higher
- fasting blood glucose level of 110 mg/dL or higher.

If you meet the criteria for metabolic syndrome, consider it a wake-up call to change your habits. (See "10 steps to a longer and healthier life," page 20.)

**Inflammation.** Mounting evidence that inflammation is a major player in atherosclerosis has led researchers to develop a test for a marker of blood vessel inflammation. For years, doctors have measured blood levels of C-reactive protein (CRP), an indicator of inflammation, to monitor diseases such as pneumonia, rheumatoid arthritis, and lupus. However, a high-sensitivity test, called hsCRP, is more specific to blood vessels.

## ▶ How to reduce your risk of heart disease

✔ Get active (see "Keep moving," page 20).

✔ Keep your cholesterol in check (see "Unfavorable cholesterol profile," page 6).

✔ Improve your diet (see "Adopt a healthy eating pattern," page 22).

✔ Keep your blood pressure within healthy limits (see "High blood pressure," page 6).

✔ Watch your weight (see "Mind your BMI," page 23).

✔ Reduce blood sugar, if it's high (see "Diabetes," page 15).

✔ Shun cigarettes (see page 20).

Studies show that people with the highest CRP levels are about twice as likely to develop coronary artery disease and suffer a heart attack or other cardiac event as people with the lowest levels. As a result, hsCRP test results are now increasingly used along with other markers (such as cholesterol and blood pressure) to estimate cardiovascular risk.

Official guidelines for hsCRP testing are still evolving, since it is not yet clear what CRP target levels should be for women of different ages and ethnicities. For now, levels below 1 mg/dL are considered low risk; 1 to 3 mg/dL, average risk; and over 3 mg/dL, high risk. The test should be reserved as a tiebreaker when considering whether a woman should take medication to reduce her overall cardiovascular risk.

**Anemia.** Anemia is a condition in which a person does not have enough red blood cells. These cells carry oxygen to your tissues, so anemia can leave you feeling tired or weak as it reduces the heart muscle's oxygen supply. The WISE study, funded by the National Institutes of Health, determined that cardiovascular outcomes are worse for anemic women than for women with normal levels of hemoglobin (the oxygen-carrying molecule in red blood cells). In older women, anemia commonly results from inflammation; decreased iron absorption due to a reduction in gastric acid; declining kidney function, which slows hemoglobin production; or certain medications, including cephalosporins, penicillin, and nonsteroidal anti-inflammatory drugs.

**Overweight and obesity.** Not only is obesity closely linked to high blood pressure, unfavorable cholesterol levels, lack of exercise, and diabetes, but it also increases your risk for heart disease independent of these other conditions. All forms of obesity are bad for health, but excessive upper-body fat (the "apple" shape) is more dangerous to the heart than lower-body obesity (the "pear" shape).

**Sedentary lifestyle.** The absence of any leisure physical activity roughly doubles the risk for coronary artery disease, making it as risky as smoking, high cholesterol, or high blood pressure. Regular physical activity prevents heart disease because it also helps to reduce many coronary risk factors. Exercise burns body fat and raises HDL cholesterol levels. It also lowers triglycerides, blood sugar, and blood pressure. In addition, it helps alleviate mental stress, which can be a trigger for heart problems. Sitting for hours at a time can increase the risk of cardiovascular disease and diabetes, even for people who exercise. If you're working on a project or have a job that keeps you chairbound, it's a good idea to stand—and even better to take a short walk—every 30 minutes or so.

**Psychological factors.** Your mental health can also affect your heart disease risk in a number of different ways.

- **Stress.** Stress can raise blood pressure, reduce blood flow to the heart, decrease the heart's pumping ability, trigger abnormal pumping rhythms, and activate the blood's clotting system and its inflammatory response. Surprisingly, research indicates that chronic stress may be more harmful to your heart than major life changes. For instance, one large study found that women who cared for a disabled spouse for at least nine hours a week faced a higher chance of having a heart attack or dying from heart disease than women without such spousal responsibilities.

- **Depression.** The relationship between depression and heart disease is a two-way street. Depression roughly doubles your risk of developing coronary artery disease, according to one review article. Other studies show that people who already have heart disease are three times as likely to be depressed as other people. As many as one in five heart attack survivors develops depression. And depression is an independent risk factor for a subsequent heart attack in people who've already had one. This may be in part because people who are depressed are less likely to take proper care of themselves—by quitting smoking, taking medications, or exercising—even after a heart attack.

- **Hostility and anger.** People who are habitually angry are two to three times as likely to have a heart attack or other cardiac event as others, according to one review article.
- **Social isolation.** Evidence shows that men and women who live alone are significantly more likely to have a heart attack or die suddenly from one. On the flip side, older adults with a strong network of friends are significantly less likely to die over a 10-year period than those without robust social support.

# Stroke

Strokes occur when part of the brain does not get enough blood, most often as the result of a blockage in a blood vessel. Strokes are not an equal-opportunity health crisis. About 425,000 of the 795,000 people who have strokes each year in the United States are women, and more women die of strokes than men do. Moreover, research shows a worrisome gender difference even in midlife. Women ages 45 to 54 are more than twice as likely as men the same age to suffer a stroke.

Women are thought to have a higher rate of strokes because of two gender-specific factors—hormonal changes during pregnancy and menopause, and the use of birth control pills. Women also have a higher rate of migraine headaches than men do. Migraines are associated with an increased risk of strokes. Moreover, later in life, women tend to have higher blood pressure than men do, also increasing stroke risk.

Stroke is often called a "brain attack." Just as a disrupted blood flow to the heart kills heart cells, so does a blockage in blood flow to the brain kill brain cells. Damage from strokes is sometimes reversible, but strokes can also result in permanent loss of the ability to move one side of the body or the loss of speech or other body functions, depending upon what area

▶ **How to reduce your risk of stroke**

- ✔ Get active (see "Keep moving," page 20).
- ✔ Keep your cholesterol in check (see "Unfavorable cholesterol profile," page 6).
- ✔ Improve your diet (see "Adopt a healthy eating pattern," page 22).
- ✔ Keep your blood pressure within healthy limits (see "High blood pressure," page 6).
- ✔ Watch your weight (see "Mind your BMI," page 23).
- ✔ Reduce blood sugar, if it's high (see "Diabetes," page 15).
- ✔ Shun cigarettes (see page 20).

of the brain is affected. The severity of the damage depends on factors such as the location of the stroke, the extent of tissue injury, and how quickly symptoms are treated. There are two basic types of strokes: ischemic and hemorrhagic.

- In ischemic strokes, which make up more than 80% of all cases, the cause is a blood clot blocking an artery supplying the brain. The clot may form in a blood vessel within the brain (thrombotic stroke), or it may form elsewhere and travel to the brain, where it lodges in a narrow vessel (embolic stroke). If the blood supply is interrupted only temporarily, so that symptoms go away in less than a day, it's called a transient ischemic attack (TIA), sometimes called a warning stroke or ministroke. A TIA must be taken seriously and treated as an emergency, because at the start, there's no way to distinguish it from a full-blown stroke. In addition, about one-third of those who experience a TIA will go on to have a full stroke, often within a year.
- In hemorrhagic strokes, which make up slightly less than 20% of cases, a blood vessel in the brain bursts. Not only are brain cells deprived of the blood supplied by the vessel, but surrounding tissue is also damaged, as leaking blood irritates brain cells and creates pressure on the brain.

Although the survival rate from strokes is increasing, female stroke survivors are likely to be more disabled and more likely to enter a nursing home than males are. One reason women fare worse than men is that on average, their first stroke happens later in life, when they are more likely to be in declining health and less likely to have someone at home to care for them. Another is that women may be less likely to acknowledge the signs of stroke and to get help as soon as men are. For that reason, stroke prevention is especially important for women.

### Risk factors

Many of the factors that put you at risk for heart disease also increase the risk of stroke; however, they are weighted somewhat differently.

**Age.** The risk of stroke increases with each decade of life.

**Family history.** Having a close relative with heart disease or a history of stroke increases stroke risk.

**Ethnicity.** Women of African American descent have a greater risk of having a stroke, and of dying from one, than white women do.

**A previous stroke or TIA.** Women who have a stroke between ages 40 and 69 have a 22% chance of having another within five years of the first. Women who have a TIA are also at greater risk of having a stroke.

**High blood pressure.** Hypertension, which is linked to ruptured blood vessels, is the most important risk factor for hemorrhagic stroke as well as a major contributor to strokes caused by blood clots.

**Smoking.** Women who smoke have an increased risk of stroke, which climbs even higher if they use oral contraceptives.

**Unfavorable cholesterol profile.** Low HDL cholesterol levels (below 40 mg/dL) are a stronger risk factor for women than for men.

**Physical inactivity.** Lack of exercise, which is directly linked to an increased risk of heart disease, contributes to obesity and other risk factors for stroke.

**Obesity and overweight.** Being overweight increases stroke risk as well as risk for heart disease.

To calculate your 10-year risk of having a stroke, go to www.health.harvard.edu/stroke-risk. Age alone is enough to elevate your risk, so as you get older, it's increasingly important to lower your other risk factors.

## Lung cancer

Lung cancer is the leading cause of cancer death in women, claiming an estimated 71,000 lives a year—roughly equal to deaths from breast, ovarian, uterine, and cervical cancers combined. Roughly 80 percent to 90 percent of lung cancer deaths are attributable to smoking or exposure to secondhand smoke, and the rate of lung cancer mirrors the rate of smoking, but with a lag of two to three decades, since it takes time for cancer to develop. The rate of new lung cancers in women peaked in 1998. Since 2002, it has fallen about 1 percent a year.

### Risk factors

Smoking, of course, leads the list of risk factors for lung cancer, but it is not the only one.

**Tobacco smoke.** Approximately 85% to 90% of people with lung cancer are present or former smokers. After World War II, women began to smoke like men—that is, they started at a young age and smoked

---

## How to recognize stroke symptoms

To help you spot a stroke, memorize the abbreviation F.A.S.T.—which stands for face, arm, speech, time.

**Face.** Smile. Does one side of your face droop?

**Arm.** Raise both arms. Does one drift down?

**Speech.** Try to talk. Are your words slurred or garbled?

**Time.** If the answer to any of the questions above is "yes," there's a high probability that you're having a stroke. Time is important, so call 911 immediately. The sooner you get to the hospital, the better the chances of recovering or minimizing the damage.

The American Stroke Association, which devised this list, also makes the information available as a smartphone app, which features a short video demonstration of the F.A.S.T. symptoms, a search function that shows nearby hospitals, and a time-stamp function that records when symptoms begin, which can aid health care workers in their treatment.

It also lists additional symptoms, which include sudden numbness, sudden confusion, sudden trouble seeing, sudden trouble walking, dizziness, or a sudden headache with no known cause.

---

## How to reduce your risk of lung cancer

✔ Shun cigarettes (see page 20).

✔ Test your house for radon and take steps to reduce it if necessary.

✔ Avoid exposure to environmental toxins if at all possible.

more heavily. Because it can take decades for lung cancer to develop, a rise in the cancer rate among women did not show up immediately, but it soared later. In the 1960s, a woman's risk of dying of lung cancer was only three times higher if she was a smoker versus a nonsmoker. Today, that risk is 25 times higher, as detailed in a 2013 *New England Journal of Medicine* study that tracked trends in smoking-related deaths over the past 50 years. Cigarette smoking among women has now declined to approximately 15% in the United States. But passive smoking also makes you susceptible; living with a smoker can increase your risk 20% to 30%.

**Radon.** Exposure to the radioactive gas emitted by uranium as it decays is the second leading cause of

### Finding lung cancer early

In 2013, the U.S. Preventive Services Task Force published new screening guidelines for lung cancer. (Screening means testing for hidden disease in people who don't have any outward signs or symptoms.) The new guidelines recommend annual screening with low-dose computed tomography (LDCT) if you're between the ages of 55 and 80 and are a heavy smoker or a former heavy smoker who quit within the past 15 years. Heavy smoking is defined as smoking at least a pack a day for at least 30 years, or two packs a day for 15 years.

These guidelines are based on a large study suggesting that for heavy smokers, annual screening can lower the risk of dying of lung cancer by 20%. The test has the potential to find lung tumors early, when they're more likely to be successfully treated. But CT scans have drawbacks: they expose you to radiation, and they often detect abnormalities that aren't cancer but must still be assessed with additional scans, biopsies, or surgeries, which carry their own risks. For these reasons, you should talk with your clinician before deciding whether to undergo CT screening for lung cancer.

lung cancer deaths. Living in homes with radon levels above 4 picocuries/liter—the level deemed safe by the Environmental Protection Agency (EPA)—may increase the risk for lung cancer. You can find information on testing your home and order test kits from the EPA website, at www.epa.gov/radon.

**Environmental toxins.** Asbestos, organic chemicals, tar, soot, or air pollution has been implicated in lung cancer development, but the relative risk posed by each of these substances hasn't been established.

**Genetics.** People with a first-degree relative who developed lung cancer, especially at an early age, may be at elevated risk.

# Chronic obstructive pulmonary disease

Chronic bronchitis and emphysema, the lung diseases grouped together under the term chronic obstructive pulmonary disease (COPD), develop gradually over many years, as the airways become narrowed and the lungs lose their ability to expand and contract effectively when you breathe. In most people with COPD, these problems stem from inflammation that occurs when something—most often cigarette smoke—irritates the respiratory tract.

The irritant can damage the cells that line the airways and can cause changes in the glands and cells that normally produce small amounts of mucus to lubricate the airway walls. In response, the body unleashes a flood of inflammatory cells, which start a chemical cascade that further damages the airways and degrades lung tissue. The cells infiltrate the walls of the airways and trigger the production of mucus inside the airways, leaving less room for air to pass. They also prompt the release of enzymes that eventually break down the lung tissue. By the time you notice symptoms—namely, coughing and breathlessness—50% to 70% of lung tissue may be lost.

### Risk factors

The following factors make a person more likely to develop COPD.

**Smoking.** COPD is more than four times as prevalent among smokers as among nonsmokers, affecting

✔ Shun cigarettes (see page 20).

✔ Reduce your exposure to environmental toxins and fumes.

about 14% of the former and just 3% of the latter. In addition, smokers are 10 to 12 times more likely to die from COPD. An intriguing question is why even more smokers don't get COPD. The fact that a relatively small percentage of smokers is affected strongly suggests that genetic factors play a role.

**Other irritants.** Exposure to air pollution, toxic fumes, industrial smoke, and dust for many years also increases risk of COPD.

**Genetics.** Alpha-1-antitrypsin (A1AT) deficiency is an inherited condition involving a defect in the gene that controls the production of A1AT, a protein that neutralizes a protease that degrades lung tissue. When the gene is defective, the level of A1AT is about 15% of normal, giving proteases free rein to wreak havoc on the lungs. In all, A1AT deficiency causes 3% of cases of emphysema. Smokers who have the genetic defect are almost certain to get emphysema.

# Alzheimer's disease

Alzheimer's disease exacts a disproportionately heavy toll on women. About two-thirds of the five million Americans with Alzheimer's are women. Moreover, women make up 60% to 70% of caregivers for people with Alzheimer's.

It's not clear what sequence of events in the brain causes Alzheimer's to develop. According to the leading theory, small fragments of soluble beta-amyloid protein in the brain may be the toxic factor, as well as another protein called tau; these trigger a series of biochemical changes leading to the death of brain cells. Two telltale signs of the disease are plaques made of beta-amyloid and neurofibrillary tangles made of tau—abnormalities visible in microscopic examination of the brain during an autopsy.

Whatever the cause of Alzheimer's, the results are clear. The brain gradually loses cells (neurons) and the connections (synapses) between neurons that enable memory and other mental functions. Levels of brain chemicals known as neurotransmitters, which carry complex messages among billions of neurons, also decrease. In advanced Alzheimer's disease, the dramatic loss of neurons causes the brain to shrink.

After the symptoms first appear, people live anywhere from two to 20 years in an increasingly dependent state that exacts a staggering emotional, physical, and economic toll on families.

There is no cure for Alzheimer's, but early diagnosis can still make a difference. Drugs are available that may temporarily stabilize or slow the progression of cognitive symptoms. These medications work best in the early stages of the disease.

▶ **How to reduce your risk of Alzheimer's**

✔ Keep your blood pressure within healthy limits (see "High blood pressure," page 6).

✔ Keep your cholesterol in check (see "Unfavorable cholesterol profile," page 6).

✔ Watch your weight (see "Mind your BMI," page 23).

✔ Avoid diabetes (see page 15).

✔ Sidestep a sedentary lifestyle (see "Keep moving," page 20).

✔ Wear a helmet while riding a bike.

## Risk factors

Some of the risk factors for Alzheimer's, such as age and genetics, are things you cannot change. But according to a 2011 review in the journal *Lancet Neurology*, up to half of cases are potentially attributable to lifestyle factors that a person can modify, including smoking, midlife obesity, physical inactivity, and failure to control heart disease.

**Age.** Risk usually rises after age 65 and doubles every five years thereafter.

**Genetics.** Heredity is a decisive factor in only a small number of families, primarily those with early-onset Alzheimer's, in which the disease begins before age 60, striking people in their 40s and 50s. Mutations in three genes are known to cause this type of

Alzheimer's: the amyloid precursor protein (APP) gene, presenilin 1, and presenilin 2. All three genetic mutations increase the production of beta-amyloid, which is deposited in the plaques found in Alzheimer's disease.

In late-onset Alzheimer's, the more common form of the disease, the genetic link is not as strong. But APOE4—one of several alleles (versions) of the gene that encodes for apolipoprotein E, a key protein in several biological processes—influences susceptibility to Alzheimer's. APOE4 has been found in about 40% of people with late-onset Alzheimer's. An estimated 25% to 30% of the population carries APOE4 (see "APOE: To test or not to test?" above).

**Cardiovascular risk factors.** Many studies show that the same things that harm the heart and blood vessels also increase the risk of Alzheimer's disease and vascular dementia. These include high blood pressure, high cholesterol, obesity, and smoking. All of these factors also increase the risk of stroke, which can be a direct cause of dementia.

**Diabetes.** People with diabetes are twice as likely to develop Alzheimer's disease as those without diabetes. Research indicates that this increase in risk may reflect a shared mechanism—a resistance of cells to the effects of insulin, the hormone that enables cells in the body to use glucose.

**Head injury.** The microscopic changes in the brains of boxers and football players with dementia resemble those in Alzheimer's disease—especially the presence of neurofibrillary tangles. The observation has led researchers to wonder if brain injury might be a factor in the disease.

**Sedentary lifestyle.** A meta-analysis of 16 prospective studies on the association between physical activity and dementia found that participants who were most active had a 45% lower risk of Alzheimer's compared with those who were least active.

# Accidents

The leading killer in women under 35, accidents are one cause of death that actually declines with passing years. Yet more than 40,000 women die annually from unintentional injuries (the CDC's term for accidents). Three types of accidents—falls, motor vehicle accidents, and poisonings—account for about two-thirds of these deaths.

**Falls.** The leading cause of home-injury fatalities, falls were responsible for the deaths of about 15,000 women in 2013. The risk of falling, and of incurring a head injury or fracture in a fall, increases with age.

**Traffic accidents.** Fatal motor vehicle accidents are about three times more likely among men than women, primarily when men are behind the wheel. However, in 2014, 9,438 women—including 1,466 pedestrians—were killed in traffic accidents.

**Poisoning.** People tend to equate poison with toxic chemicals, but alcohol and prescription drugs have emerged as the leading causes of poisoning

> ## How to reduce your risk of an accidental injury
>
> ✔ Don't drink and drive.
>
> ✔ Buckle up when you drive, and practice commonsense precautions, such as driving within the speed limit and not using your cellphone.
>
> ✔ Tell your doctor about all the medications you are taking, so you can make substitutions for those most likely to affect your balance and avoid accidental drug interactions or overdoses.
>
> ✔ At home, remove tripping hazards such as loose rugs, install handrails or grab bars if necessary, and ensure that you have proper lighting so you can see obstacles clearly.

death in women. Drug overdoses claimed the lives of 18,243 women in 2014.

# Breast cancer

The statistical picture of breast cancer has brightened, thanks to advances in diagnosis and treatment. More tumors are being caught at an early stage, and the death rate has dropped. A marked decline in the incidence of breast cancer since 2003 has been tied to women's abandonment of long-term postmenopausal hormone therapy.

You can estimate your risk for breast cancer by using the National Cancer Institute's online calculator, at www.cancer.gov/bcrisktool.

### Risk factors

Since the early 1990s, researchers have located the genes responsible for the most devastating hereditary

---

### Figure 2: Do digital mammograms make a difference?

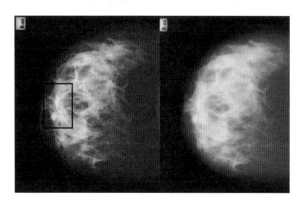

On mammograms, fat looks dark gray, and breast tissue, which is denser, shows as white. Abnormalities, such as microcalcifications and lumps, also appear white, making it difficult to distinguish them from the surrounding tissue.

In the digital image (left), a cancerous mass can be seen as solid white (boxed in red), just behind the nipple. On a standard mammogram of the same breast (right), the tumor is harder to spot. However, studies have not shown that digital mammography is more effective at detecting cancer, except perhaps in women who have dense breasts and are younger than 50. If you are older than 50, the main advantage may be that the digital mammograms can be stored and retrieved electronically, which makes long-distance consultations with specialists easier.

---

### ▶ How to reduce your risk of breast cancer

✔ Improve your diet (see "Adopt a healthy eating pattern," page 22).

✔ Watch your weight (see "Mind your BMI," page 23).

✔ Stay active (see "Keep moving," page 20).

✔ Follow mammography screening advice (see "When do you need a mammogram?" on page 15).

✔ Minimize your exposure to estrogen (see "Estrogen exposure," below).

✔ Don't drink more than one alcoholic beverage a day (see "Lift a glass, but only one," page 24).

---

forms of the disease and have identified risk factors that are within most women's power to change.

**Family history.** Hereditary breast cancers account for approximately 5% to 10% of all cases. However, inheriting a mutation in either the BRCA1 or BRCA2 gene can raise breast cancer risk by 45% to 65%. Women of Ashkenazi Jewish heritage are about five times more likely than other women to have one of these mutations. If you've tested positive for either one, you may want to ask your doctors about options for risk reduction, including surgical removal of the ovaries (if premenopausal), bilateral mastectomy, or use of the drugs tamoxifen and raloxifene.

**Estrogen exposure.** Because estrogen fuels breast cell growth, the longer your ovaries were producing estrogen, the greater your risk of breast cancer. Any of these conditions means greater estrogen exposure—menstruation before age 12, menopause after 55, pregnancy after 35, or no pregnancies. Postmenopausal hormone therapy adds to the risk.

**Breast history.** Dense breasts, which have more fibrous or glandular tissue and less fat, may increase your risk, as they can indicate a propensity for tissue to proliferate. Prior breast biopsies, especially those that revealed precancerous abnormalities, such as lobular carcinoma in situ, are also linked to a higher risk. And having had one cancerous breast tumor increases the risk of another malignancy.

**Radiation therapy.** Chest radiation to treat cancer increases the risk of developing breast cancer later in life, especially if you had the radiation during

## When do you need a mammogram?

In 2015, both the American Cancer Society (ACS) and the U.S. Preventive Services Task Force (USPSTF) revised their guidelines for breast cancer screening. Expert panels selected by each organization reviewed reams of evidence to weigh the benefits and risks of mammography. The two sets of guidelines are similar but not identical (see Table 2, below). The ACS recommends routine screening beginning at age 45, while the USPSTF recommends starting routine screening at 50. The USPSTF also concluded that screening every two years had similar benefits as annual screening—and with fewer harms. (The particular drawbacks of screening are different at different times of life. False alarms are more common for women ages 40 to 49, whereas unnecessary treatment is a greater concern for women in the older age groups.)

Because there is no evidence that breast self-exams save lives, neither the ACS or the USPSTF guidelines advise women to do them. Instead, you can use breast self-awareness—being aware of what your normal breasts are like.

### Other breast imaging tests

**Ultrasound.** If your doctor feels a lump in your breast, or if a mammogram detects one, an ultrasound might be suggested to determine if the lump is solid (which could be cancer) or fluid-filled (which is usually a benign cyst). Ultrasound may also be used in addition to mammography for some women with dense breast tissue.

**Magnetic resonance imaging.** This test is recommended for women at high risk (greater than 20% lifetime risk) for breast cancer, such as those with a BRCA gene mutation, those who have received radiation for Hodgkin's lymphoma, or a combination of risk factors on a breast cancer risk assessment tool.

**Tomosynthesis (3D mammography).** In this newer form of digital mammography, the machine takes many low-dose x-rays at multiple angles as it moves over the compressed breast. The images can then be combined into a three-dimensional picture that allows a radiologist to differentiate a tumor from superimposed tissue. This reduces a woman's chance of being called back for more imaging tests. However, the procedure uses more radiation than traditional mammography and is not widely available. Newer tomosynthesis techniques lower the radiation dose to slightly above that of a conventional mammogram, but most facilities have not yet upgraded because of the high cost. Tomosynthesis shows promise in screening women with dense breast tissue and high risk for breast cancer, but its role in screening and diagnosis still remains unclear.

### Table 2: Mammography guidelines for average-risk women based on age

| AGE | ACS | USPSTF |
|---|---|---|
| 45 to 49 | Annual screening | No routine screening |
| 50 to 54 | Annual screening | Biennial screening |
| 55 and older | Biennial screening as long as a woman is healthy and has a life expectancy of at least 10 years | Biennial screening through age 74; insufficient evidence to recommend for or against screening for women 75 and older |

*Sources: American Cancer Society; U.S. Preventive Services Task Force.*

puberty. In women who have a BRCA gene mutation, the risk is amplified, especially for chest radiation received before age 20.

**Obesity.** Probably because estrogen is produced by body fat in addition to the ovaries, obesity raises the risk of breast cancer, especially after menopause.

**Alcohol use.** Alcohol has also been shown to increase circulating estrogen levels, so breast cancer risk increases with every drink taken. Although the risk is slight for women who limit their daily consumption to one drink (see Figure 5, page 24), it mounts steadily with greater intake.

**Lack of exercise.** Growing evidence is implicating inactivity as a contributing factor to breast cancer.

## Diabetes

Blood sugar (glucose) is the fuel that the body uses for energy. Diabetes develops when the body's ability to turn glucose into energy breaks down and blood glucose levels rise to dangerously high levels. Left untreated or poorly managed, it can lead to serious long-term complications, including kidney failure, amputation, and blindness.

There are two types of diabetes. About 5% to 10% of people with diabetes are diagnosed with type 1 diabetes, which develops after the body's immune system mistakenly destroys cells in the pancreas, so that this organ can no longer produce the insulin necessary to metabolize blood sugar. This form of the disease usually develops before age 20.

Far more common—and preventable—is type 2 diabetes, which affects 90% to 95% of people with diabetes. It tends to occur in adults over 40, and its incidence increases with age, although recent increases in obesity have put younger people at greater risk as well.

## ▶ How to reduce your risk of type 2 diabetes

✔ Watch your weight (see "Mind your BMI," page 23).

✔ Boost your activity level. Regular exercise protects you, even if you don't lose weight (see "Keep moving," page 20).

✔ Improve your diet (see "Adopt a healthy eating pattern," page 22).

Type 2 diabetes takes years to develop. The process begins when cells of the body become less responsive to insulin. To keep blood sugar levels under control, the pancreas compensates by pumping out more insulin. At first, blood sugar levels stay within a normal range. But for some, the insulin-producing cells eventually fail to keep up with the increased demand. As a result, blood sugar levels rise, resulting first in a problem known as prediabetes, and finally progressing to full-blown diabetes.

A doctor generally diagnoses the disease when fasting blood sugar is 126 mg/dL or higher on two separate tests; when an oral glucose tolerance test shows a blood sugar reading of 200 mg/dL or more two hours after drinking a sugary liquid; or when HbA1c, a measure of average blood sugar over the previous two to three months, is 6.5% or higher. You may also have symptoms of high blood sugar, such as blurry vision, excessive thirst, and frequent urination.

## Risk factors

Reducing controllable risk factors can often prevent type 2 diabetes from developing.

**Age.** Predominantly a disease of later life, type 2 diabetes generally develops after age 40. People over age 65 are at particularly high risk.

**Family history.** Having a first-degree relative with diabetes raises the risk. If one of your parents was diagnosed with type 2 diabetes before age 50, your risk of getting the disease is roughly one in seven. If your parent was diagnosed after age 50, the risk is about one in 13. If both of your parents developed type 2 diabetes, your odds are about one in two.

**Ethnicity.** The disease is far more common among African Americans, Hispanics, Asian Americans, Pacific Islanders, and Native Americans than among whites.

**Obesity or overweight.** Of the more than one million Americans who develop diabetes annually, about 80% are overweight or obese. The distribution of body fat seems to be important. People who tend to store fat in the abdominal area are more likely to become diabetic than those who put it on around the hips.

**High blood pressure.** Risk increases at blood pressure levels of 140/90 mm Hg and above.

**Sedentary lifestyle.** Exercising fewer than three days a week puts you at increased risk.

**Polycystic ovary syndrome (PCOS).** Women with PCOS usually have insulin resistance or other diabetes risk factors.

**Gestational diabetes.** This form of the disease begins during pregnancy and usually resolves after delivery, but many women with this problem later develop diabetes, usually five to 10 years after the pregnancy.

**Prediabetes.** This is defined as having fasting blood glucose levels of 100 to 125 mg/dL or oral glucose tolerance test levels of 140 to 199 mg/dL.

**Medication use.** Some drugs can increase insulin resistance or decrease insulin secretion. Either way, the result is higher levels of glucose in the bloodstream. These medications include diuretics, corticosteroids, beta blockers, and a class of drugs called atypical or second-generation antipsychotics, originally developed to treat schizophrenia.

# Influenza and pneumonia

Microbes are ever-present among us. While some of them, particularly the bacteria that inhabit the gastro-intestinal system, coexist peacefully and productively with their human hosts, others cause diseases, including influenza and pneumonia.

Flu is caused by a highly infectious respiratory virus and is usually spread from one person to the next when the infected person coughs or sneezes. (Droplets containing the flu virus can travel as much as six feet, so you don't need to be standing right next to someone to become infected.) Less often, you can become infected after touching a contaminated surface such as a doorknob. In healthy people, flu can hit with a wallop, causing fever, chills, fatigue, maybe a headache, muscle aches, or sore throat. In older adults or people with other medical conditions, flu can be deadly. One of the challenges in fighting flu is that viruses mutate so rapidly that older vaccines don't necessarily work against them. That's why the flu shot has to be reformulated every year.

Pneumonia also develops because of a respiratory infection, although the cause can be a virus, bacteria, or even an inhaled chemical. There are two main types of pneumonia. Viral pneumonia is caused by respiratory viruses such as the flu virus. Bacterial pneumonia can be triggered directly by any one of dozens of bacteria, or it may emerge as a complication of flu or another viral infection. However it develops, pneumonia causes fever, chills, cough, and difficulty breathing—and sometimes death. In women, pneumonia accounts for more than 28,000 deaths annually, and influenza less than 2,000.

## ▶ How to reduce your risk of flu or pneumonia

✔ Get vaccinated (see Table 4, page 26).

✔ Wash your hands or use hand sanitizers frequently throughout the day.

✔ Shun cigarettes (see page 20).

✔ If you do get the flu, see your doctor so you can get prompt treatment and avoid having it turn into pneumonia.

## Risk factors

Being aware of the following risk factors can help you avoid catching flu or pneumonia.

**Smoking.** Smokers are more likely to get the flu than nonsmokers—as are people exposed to second-hand smoke.

**Crowded and close environments.** Spending time in places like nursing homes, schools, shopping malls, and movie theaters increases the risk of contracting the flu virus.

**Age.** Children ages 2 and under face the highest risk, followed by people 65 and older.

**Existing medical conditions.** Cancer, neuromuscular diseases, chronic pulmonary conditions, and cardiovascular diseases, as well as immunosuppressive disorders and drug therapy that can suppress the immune system, all increase the risk of getting the flu.

**Dental plaque.** Even the bacteria that inhabit dental plaque can migrate to the lungs to cause pneumonia. The risk is greatest in people on ventilators and in nursing homes.

## Flu and pneumonia vaccine recommendations

Vaccines significantly reduce the risk of pneumonia and influenza. A pneumococcal polysaccharide vaccine—pneumococcal 13-valent conjugate (PCV13), which offers protection from pneumococcal pneumonia, blood infection, and meningitis—is recommended at age 65. It is to be followed by a second vaccine—pneumococcal 23-valent polysaccharide (PPSV23)—a year or more later. Both vaccines are also advised for younger people who have chronic organ disease or compromised immunity.

The seasonal flu shot, containing killed flu virus, is recommended for all adults. A higher dose of the vaccine is advised for people over 65.

# Colorectal cancer

The third leading cause of cancer deaths, most colorectal cancers arise from lesions on the intestinal lining called adenomatous polyps. The progression from precancerous polyp to full-blown cancer is believed to take 10 years or more, though. Screening allows physicians to remove polyps before they become cancerous and to identify cancer early, when it's most treatable.

For women at average risk, colonoscopy is recommended as a screening test at age 50 and then every decade thereafter. (If you have a family history of colorectal cancer, inflammatory bowel disease, or other factors, you may need more frequent screening.) During a colonoscopy, a gastroenterologist examines the lining of the colon with a lighted scope, looking for cancerous lesions and polyps. There are other screening methods—fecal occult blood testing, flexible sigmoidoscopy, CT colonography (virtual colonoscopy), and a stool test for DNA shed by colorectal cancers. However, traditional colonoscopy is preferred because it checks the entire colon, detects the most polyps and lesions, and allows the doctor to biopsy or remove polyps and lesions during the procedure. Colonoscopy is particularly important for women, who are more likely to have polyps or lesions deeper in the ascending colon, the area at the farthest reach of the colonoscope. In contrast, sigmoidoscopy examines only the first third of the colon.

### ▶ How to reduce your risk of colorectal cancer

✔ Undergo periodic screening for colorectal cancer (see Table 3, page 26).

✔ Limit consumption of red meat and processed meats (see "Adopt a healthy eating pattern," page 22).

✔ Shun cigarettes (see page 20).

### Risk factors

Colorectal cancer is associated with a range of characteristics, conditions, and habits, as follows.

**Age.** More than 90% of colon cancers occur in people over age 50.

**Family history.** Having at least one first-degree relative with colon cancer doubles your risk of colon cancer. Two rare, inherited syndromes also raise your risk. One, called familial adenomatous polyposis, accounts for just 1% of all colon cancers—but nearly everyone who carries genetic mutations for it develops

cancer by age 40 unless they have preventive surgery to remove the colon. The other, hereditary nonpolyposis colorectal cancer (also known as Lynch syndrome), increases lifetime colon cancer risk as much 80%, although fewer than 5% of all colon cancers result from this syndrome.

**Personal history of polyps.** Although most polyps do not develop into cancer, people who have had polyps removed in a colonoscopy are at a higher risk and may require more frequent colonoscopies than people at average risk.

**History of inflammatory bowel disease (IBD).** Ulcerative colitis and Crohn's disease increase risk up to five times; however, more than 90% of people with IBD do not get colon cancer.

**Diet.** Research suggests that people who eat diets rich in red meat have higher colon cancer rates compared with those whose diets contain little or no red meat. Even worse are cured and processed meats (such as hot dogs, sausage, salami, ham, bacon, and jerky). In 2015, the World Health Organization classified cured and processed meats as a Group 1 carcinogen, meaning that there is now sufficient evidence to state that they raise the risk of cancer, in this case colon cancer—though the overall risk they pose is low compared with, say, the risk that smoking poses for lung cancer.

**Sedentary lifestyle.** Several studies have linked a lack of exercise and sedentary behavior to a higher risk of colon cancer. One such study found double the risk of certain forms of the disease among people who spent 10 or more years in sedentary jobs (such as computer workers), compared with people who spent no time in sedentary work.

## Ovarian cancer

Although it is not in the top 10 list of the most common cancers, ovarian cancer is responsible for more deaths in women than other reproductive system malignancies. It is also one of the most feared cancers, because it often is not detected until the disease has spread elsewhere in the body (metastasized). At that point, it becomes difficult to treat. However, there are ways that you can reduce your risk if you have a strong genetic or family history. Emerging data suggest that ovarian cancer starts in the fallopian tubes, and risk-reducing surgery to remove the tubes and ovaries can be offered for women who are done with childbearing. Also, you might catch ovarian cancer while it is still treatable if you see the doctor for subtle warning signs, including abdominal pain or bloating, pelvic pain, difficulty eating or feeling full quickly, and urgent or frequent urination.

## Risk factors

The following are linked to an increased risk.

**Age.** The median age of diagnosis is 63.

**Heredity.** A family or personal history of ovarian or breast cancer indicates an increased risk. Women with a BRCA1 mutation have a 35% to 70% higher lifetime risk than women without the mutation; for BRCA2, the increase in risk is 10% to 30% by age 70. Another genetic syndrome, hereditary nonpolyposis colorectal cancer, has also been associated with endometrial and ovarian cancer.

**Postmenopausal estrogen use.** Five or more years of estrogen as postmenopausal hormone therapy, without concurrent use of a progestin, has been shown to increase risk in several large studies.

**Overweight or obesity.** A large observational study indicated that a body mass index (BMI) of 30 or greater increases the risk of ovarian cancer by 80% in postmenopausal women who have never taken hormones. You can find your BMI by entering your height and weight into the online calculator at www.health.harvard.edu/BMI.

**Factors that reduce risk.** Pregnancy, the long-term use of oral contraceptives, tubal ligation, removal of the fallopian tubes, and hysterectomy are all factors that decrease the risk for most women, but experts agree that a hysterectomy should only be performed for medical reasons unrelated to ovarian cancer prevention. With hysterectomy, the risk reduction is greatest if the ovaries and fallopian tubes are also removed, along with the uterus. With tubal ligation, risk reduction is greatest if the tubes are also removed. ♥

# 10 steps to a longer and healthier life

**D**on't dwell on the risk factors you can't control; instead, focus your efforts on the things you can do to help feel strong and healthy during the second half of your life. Risk reduction has a lot in common with one-stop shopping: it's possible to reduce your risk for many major degenerative diseases at once by following the advice in this chapter.

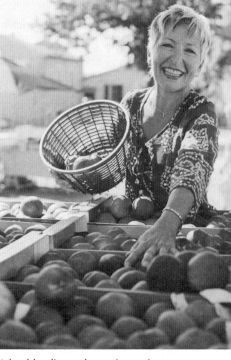

A healthy diet and exercise regimen can go a long way to reducing your risks for multiple chronic diseases at once. Think of it as one-stop shopping for your health.

### ① Shun cigarettes

If you smoke, quit. There are few things you can do that will have such immediate and lasting benefits as giving up smoking. In 20 minutes, your heart rate will fall. By the next day, you'll have cleared the excess carbon monoxide from your blood. Within months, you'll be breathing more easily and coughing much less. Over the years, your risk for lung cancer, stroke, and heart disease will drop by at least half. And in 15 years, you'll have erased your excess risk for heart disease.

In addition, separate yourself from smokers. Long-term exposure to other people's smoke is a weaker, but still noteworthy, risk factor. If you're a nonsmoker, become a nag. Let the smokers in your circle of friends and family know that you would like them to quit, and encourage them in their efforts. Be patient. Only 4% to 7% of smokers are able to quit without aids like nicotine replacement products or medical help, and only one-quarter to one-third who use any quit-smoking medicine stay smoke-free for more than six months. It usually takes many attempts before a person is successful at quitting.

### ② Keep moving

Lack of physical activity is an independent risk factor for nearly all of the diseases that are most likely to kill or disable you. In the long-running Framingham Heart Study, sedentary women died a year and a half earlier than those who were moderately active. Women who were very active enjoyed three-and-a-half more years than their sedentary counterparts.

Regular moderate exercise can help to protect you against the following problems:

**Heart disease and stroke.** Regular exercise helps you strike a healthier balance of blood lipids (HDL, LDL, and triglycerides) and helps arteries retain resilience despite the effects of aging. It reduces blood pressure, which in turn lowers the risk not just of heart disease, but also of stroke and kidney failure. Exercising regularly may also promote the

© Digital Vision | Thinkstock

growth of collateral arteries, small blood vessels feeding the heart. Even if you already have heart disease, exercise lowers your chances of dying from it.

**Cancer.** Exercise reduces the risk of cancers of the colon, breast, and endometrium. By helping you attain a healthy weight, exercise also lessens your risk for other cancers in which obesity is a factor (see "Mind your BMI," page 23).

**Diabetes.** Exercise pares excess weight, modestly lowers blood sugar levels, and boosts sensitivity to insulin, reducing your risk of developing type 2 diabetes. If you already have diabetes, exercise helps control blood sugar.

**Osteoporosis.** When combined with bone-saving medications (if necessary), weight-bearing exercise—such as walking, running, or classic strength training, and even some yoga routines—helps ward off bone loss.

**Arthritis.** Exercise helps protect joints by easing swelling, pain, and fatigue and by keeping cartilage healthy. Strong muscles support joints and lighten the load upon them. Exercise may limit and even reverse knee problems by helping to control weight.

**Accidents.** Activities like stretching, yoga, and tai chi and exercises to increase core strength extend your range of motion and enhance balance, which helps prevent falls and other accidents.

**Depression and anxiety.** Exercise lifts spirits by releasing

## How much exercise is enough?

According to guidelines from the U.S. Department of Health and Human Services (HHS), every adult should get at least 150 minutes of moderate aerobic activity a week (for example, walking at a rate of 3 to 5 mph) or 75 minutes of higher-intensity activity (5 mph or more). The sessions should be at least 10 minutes long and may combine moderate and vigorous activities. In addition, adults should engage in at least two sessions of strengthening exercises a week.

But the HHS committee found that you can get even greater health benefits and more effective weight control when you reach twice the recommended weekly amount—that is, 300 minutes of moderate activity, 150 minutes of vigorous activity, or a combination of the two—and more than that may be better still. Research suggests that women who meet the 300-minutes-per-week goal have high aerobic fitness, which translates to a lower body mass index, better cholesterol levels, lower blood pressure, and fewer chronic conditions like diabetes and heart disease. They also appear to be less likely to die from breast cancer. But ramp up slowly, to reduce the likelihood of injury. Once you're routinely logging the basic recommended levels of aerobic activity, start to add a few minutes a day.

The HHS guidelines emphasize that people with chronic medical conditions and disabilities should get just as much exercise as other adults, if possible. Speak with your health care provider about appropriate kinds and levels of exercise. The American College of Sports Medicine website also has detailed advice for people with certain chronic health conditions; you can find it at www.health.harvard.edu/exercise-is-medicine.

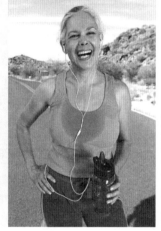

© Dave & Les Jacobs | Thinkstock

mood-elevating hormones, relieving stress, and promoting a sense of well-being. In some studies, exercising regularly has helped ease mild to moderate depression as effectively as medications; combining exercise with medications, therapy, and social engagement is even better.

**Alzheimer's disease.** Sedentary habits make you more prone to obesity, heart disease, and type 2 diabetes, all of which can raise your risk of Alzheimer's. And exercise appears to benefit brain function, which may help prevent or at least postpone the disease. In recent small studies, regular intensive exercise improved reasoning in women with mild cognitive impairment.

**Infections.** Exercise may boost your ability to fend off infection. In randomized trials, women who walked briskly 35 to 45 minutes a day, five days a week, for 12 to 15 weeks experienced half the cold symptoms of a sedentary group.

Additional research shows exercise prompts a modest, short-term upswing in natural killer cells and white blood cells, which help squelch infection.

### ③ Adopt a healthy eating pattern

For all the attention that has been devoted to the health benefits of "superfoods," nutritionists now emphasize that what really counts is not eating certain healthful foods from time to time, but having a healthy dietary pattern that you adhere to most of the time, day in, day out. Scores of observational studies have identified the dietary patterns that are associated with lower rates of heart disease, cancers, and dementia. To summarize this information, nutrition scientists and epidemiologists at Harvard T.H. Chan School of Public Health and Harvard Medical School have developed the Healthy Eating Plate, a dietary plan that is consistent with the 2015–2020 Dietary Guidelines for Americans (see Figure 3, below). Here is a summary of the main points:

**Fully half your plate should contain fruits and vegetables.** You can't go wrong if you aim for color and variety. The greater the variety, the greater the range of nutrients you will take in. And the pigments not only provide eye appeal; they are often antioxidants that reduce inflammation. (Note that for these purposes, potatoes—which are quick to raise blood sugar levels—don't count as vegetables.)

**A quarter of the plate should be filled with whole grains.** Whole wheat, barley, wheat berries, quinoa, oats, and brown rice are more nutritious and contain more fiber than refined grains. They have less effect on blood sugar and insulin than white bread, white rice, and other refined grains. Although whole grains may take a little longer to cook, they offer more interesting flavors and textures than their refined counterparts. If you're feeling adventuresome, you may want to try "ancient grains" like amaranth, spelt, and teff, which have been unchanged for centuries.

**The final quarter should consist of healthful sources of protein.** Fish, chicken, beans, and nuts are all healthy, versatile protein sources. They can be mixed into salads, and they pair well with vegetables on a plate. Limit red meat, which has been linked to an increased risk of cardiovascular disease and cancer, to one or two servings a week. Avoid processed meats such as bacon and sausage, which have been designated carcinogens by the World Health Organization.

**Include healthy plant oils.** Choose vegetable oils like olive, canola, sunflower, and peanut in cooking. Avoid partially hydrogenated oils, which increase the risk of cardiovascular disease; they are commonly found in nondairy creamers, packaged bakery goods,

### Figure 3: The healthy eating plate

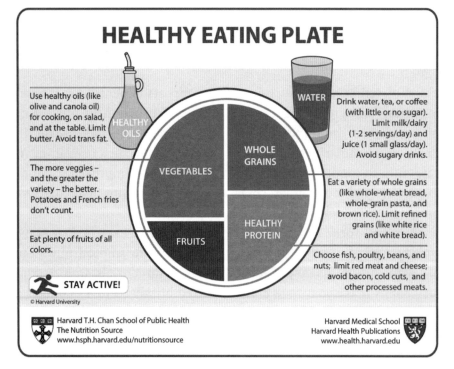

snack foods, vegetable shortenings, and stick margarines. Remember that low-fat does not mean healthy. In fact, low-fat dressings and sauces often contain more added salt and sugars than higher-fat versions.

**Drink water, coffee, or tea.** Skip sugary drinks, limit milk and dairy products to one to two servings per day, and limit fruit juice to a small glass per day.

## ④ Mind your BMI

Excess body weight increases your risk for more than 50 different health problems. These conditions include some of the leading causes of death among women—heart disease, stroke, breast cancer, and type 2 diabetes—as well as less serious ailments such as arthritic knees and gallstones.

Body mass index (BMI) uses your weight and height to gauge whether you are normal weight, overweight, or obese. You can find your BMI by entering your height and weight into the calculator at www.health.harvard.edu/BMI. A BMI of 18.5 to 24.9 is considered a normal weight. Once you reach 25, you're overweight, and anything 30 and higher is obese.

Because so many people—two in three Americans—are overweight, being heavy now seems "normal." But it's far from healthy. A Harvard study that included 120,000 women found that obesity increased the risk of diabetes 20 times and substantially boosted the risk of developing high blood pres-

sure, heart disease, stroke, or gallstones. Among people who were overweight or obese, there was a direct relationship between BMI and risk: the higher the BMI, the higher the likelihood of disease.

Studies are also linking obesity to cancer deaths. An American Cancer Society investigation that followed more than 900,000 people for 16 years suggested that overweight and obesity account for 20% of all cancer deaths in women 50 and older. Higher BMIs were associated with a higher risk of dying from cancer of the esophagus, colon and rectum, liver, gallbladder, pancreas, or kidney as well as cancer of the breast, uterus, cervix, or ovary.

Fat distribution also plays a role in health risks. While fat that accumulates in the lower body settles directly under the skin, fat in the abdomen is largely visceral, serving as padding between the organs

(see Figure 4, below). The problem with visceral fat is that it's metabolically active, producing substances that spur inflammation and increase insulin resistance. Thus an "apple" body shape—particularly a waist measurement of 35 inches or more—puts a woman at higher risk for heart disease and type 2 diabetes.

Where a woman puts on fat is influenced by heredity and hormones. A number of genes are involved in determining how many fat cells you develop and where these cells are stored. At menopause, estrogen production decreases, and there is an increase in the ratio of androgens (male hormones present in small amounts in women) to estrogen—a shift that's been linked in some studies to increased abdominal fat after menopause.

The best way to lose excess weight, wherever it is located, is to consume fewer calories than you

---

## Figure 4: Types of body fat

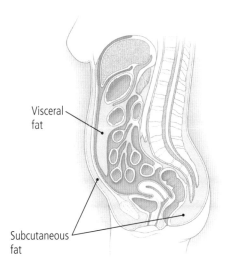

The excess pounds that tend to creep on at midlife often settle around the belly and hips. Fat that accumulates just under the skin is called subcutaneous fat. It is found in the hips, thighs, and buttocks, and between the abdominal wall and skin covering your belly. But more of the fat in the abdominal area is visceral fat. Located around the abdominal organs and inside the abdominal cavity, visceral fat appears to increase the risk of insulin resistance, which can set the stage for type 2 diabetes.

use. One way to start is to follow the exercise and dietary guidelines outlined above. Participants in the National Weight Control Registry—a database of more than 10,000 people (80% of whom are women) who have lost 30 pounds or more and kept it off for at least a year—report exercising approximately one hour a day (primarily through brisk walking); eating an average of 1,400 calories a day, with about 25% of caloric intake coming from fat; making breakfast a regular habit; and maintaining a consistent eating pattern across weekdays and weekends. They also keep close tabs on their weight, hitting the scales at least once a week.

## ⑤ Lift a glass, but only one

We toast to good health for good reason. Moderate drinking has been associated with reduced risk for heart disease and death from all causes. Alcohol of any kind increases "good" HDL cholesterol, improves insulin sensitivity, and reduces inflammation. Wine in particular contains small amounts of plant substances called flavonoids that have demonstrated anti-inflammatory and anticancer activity in laboratory experiments.

But for women, the benefits of alcohol vanish with a second drink. At more than one drink a day (see Figure 5, above right), you increase your risk of cancers of the breast, head and neck, and digestive system; high blood pressure; stroke;

### Figure 5: What is a standard drink?

- 1½ ounces (a jigger) of 80-proof liquor (bourbon, gin, rum, scotch, tequila, vodka, or whiskey)
- 2–3 ounces of fruit, coffee, chocolate, or other flavored liqueurs (cordials)
- 3 ounces of fortified wine (sherry, port, Marsala, or Madeira)
- 4–5 ounces of table wine
- 12 ounces of regular or light beer

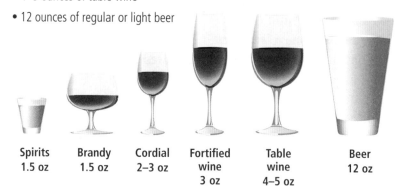

| Spirits 1.5 oz | Brandy 1.5 oz | Cordial 2–3 oz | Fortified wine 3 oz | Table wine 4–5 oz | Beer 12 oz |

and car accidents. At higher levels of consumption, the risk of pancreatic and liver disease and neurological disorders rises.

Women are more sensitive to alcohol than men, because their bodies produce less of an enzyme that breaks down alcohol in the stomach before it's absorbed into the blood. Moreover, women's bodies have a lower proportion of water (which dilutes alcohol) to fat (which retains it). Alcohol therefore remains in the female system at higher concentrations for longer periods of time and has more contact with the brain and other organs. At the same level of alcohol consumption, women become intoxicated faster, develop addiction earlier, and suffer health damage sooner than men.

Moreover, alcohol's effects become more insidious as women age, because the body's water-to-fat

ratio declines over the years. Even though you may be drinking the same amount of alcohol as when you were younger, each drink packs a bigger wallop. Women may be more likely than men to develop alcohol-related problems that are mistakenly attributed to aging, such as depression, sleep disruptions, poor eating, heart failure, and frequent falls. Women over 65 are also more likely than men to use medications for anxiety and depression, which can have dangerous interactions with alcohol.

## ⑥ Don't run up a sleep debt

Medical evidence suggests that for optimum health and function, the average adult should get seven to nine hours of sleep daily. But more than 60% of women regularly fall short of that goal. In some cases, lack of sleep results from insom-

## Sound advice for sleeping soundly

**Create a sleep sanctuary.** Reserve it for sleep and intimacy. Keep it on the cool side. Banish the television, computer, cellphone or tablet, and other diversions from that space.

**Nap only if necessary.** Night owls and shift workers are at the greatest risk for sleep debt. Napping an hour or two at the peak of sleepiness in the afternoon can help to supplement hours missed at night. But naps can also interfere with your ability to sleep at night and throw your sleep schedule into disarray.

**Avoid caffeine after noon, and go light on alcohol.** Caffeine can stay in your body for up to 12 hours. Alcohol can act as a sedative, but it also disturbs sleep.

**Get regular exercise, but not within three hours of bedtime.** Exercise acts as a short-term stimulant.

**Address a long-term debt.** If you've skimped on sleep for decades, you won't be required to put in a Rip Van Winkle–like effort to repay the hours of missed slumber. Nonetheless, it could take a few weeks to recoup your losses. Plan a vacation with a light schedule and few obligations—not a whirlwind tour of the museums of Europe or a daughter's wedding. Then, turn off the alarm clock and just sleep every night until you awake naturally. At the beginning, you may be sleeping 12 hours or more a night; by the end, you'll be getting about the amount you regularly need to awake refreshed.

**Avoid backsliding into a new debt cycle.** Once you've determined how much sleep you really need, factor it into your daily schedule. Try to go to bed and get up at the same time every day—at the very least, on weekdays. If need be, use weekends to make up for lost sleep. Rather than disrupting your sleep schedule, try taking a nap in the early afternoon to catch up; a nap of 15 to 20 minutes is best, but it should definitely not exceed an hour.

If you're able to get enough sleep but don't feel refreshed in the morning, discuss the problem with your clinician. Many common medical conditions, from depression to obstructive sleep apnea (brief cessations in breathing during sleep), could be responsible. Wearing a fitness tracker can help identify how much sleep you are actually getting by distinguishing periods of restlessness from those of deep sleep.

nia or other underlying conditions that may require medical attention. But most women with a sleep debt run it up by burning the candle at both ends—consistently failing to get to bed on time or stay there long enough. It's not hard to understand why this happens. Women often find it difficult to make up sleep lost while caring for young children and juggling family and career. Meno-

pause can add its own challenges.

Fortunately, you can repay even a chronic, longstanding sleep debt (see "Sound advice for sleeping soundly," above). Doing so can have a profound effect on your daily well-being and long-term health. Many studies show that sleep shortfalls can lead to a range of health problems, from the mild (being more likely to catch a cold)

to the more consequential (having a higher risk of high blood pressure, heart disease, obesity, and diabetes). Think of getting enough sleep—roughly seven to nine hours a night—as being just as important as eating a healthy diet and getting regular exercise.

 **Take charge of your health**

To help ensure that you're taking the best possible care of your own health, be persistent, and follow these tips:

**Form a partnership.** At midlife and beyond, good health is increasingly dependent on successful collaboration with your doctors. Since you are likely to be making more medical visits, find a primary care clinician with whom you feel comfortable. Work with your doctor to devise a schedule for screening tests and clinical exams (see Table 3, page 26). If you are prescribed medications, take them as directed; don't stray from the designated dosage without talking to your doctor. Find out what you should expect from every new medication and procedure, and let your physician know what you expect it to accomplish in return.

**Manage your medical conditions.** You may not notice any symptoms from conditions like high blood pressure, high cholesterol, diabetes, or glaucoma. But it's important to work with your doctor to keep these under control. Problems can develop for

## Table 3: Routine screening tests for women ages 50 or older

Screening is testing for diseases and conditions that may not yet be causing symptoms. If you already have a particular disease or condition—or are at high risk for one—more frequent testing may be required.

| TEST | RECOMMENDATION |
|---|---|
| Blood pressure testing | Get tested at least every two years if you have normal blood pressure (lower than 120/80). |
| BRCA risk testing | If you have family members with breast, ovarian, tubal, or peritoneal cancer, you should consider having a blood test to detect potentially harmful mutations in breast cancer susceptibility genes BRCA1 and BRCA2. |
| Breast cancer screening | Some disagreement exists over screening (see Table 2, page 15), but the USPSTF recommends a mammogram every two years from ages 50 through 74. Women 75 or older should discuss screening with their doctors. |
| Cholesterol testing | Get a cholesterol test regularly if you are at increased risk for heart disease. Ask your doctor or nurse how often you need your cholesterol tested. |
| Colorectal cancer screening | Starting at age 50, get screened for colorectal cancer. Talk to your doctor or nurse about which screening test—fecal occult blood, sigmoidoscopy, or colonoscopy—is best for you and how often you need it. |
| Diabetes screening | Get screened for diabetes if your blood pressure is higher than 135/80 or if you take medicine for high blood pressure. The National Institutes of Health also recommends screening if you are overweight or obese. |
| Hepatitis B virus testing | You may need a blood test for hepatitis B virus infection if you are at high risk for infection. |
| Hepatitis C virus testing | If you were born between 1945 and 1965, you should have a blood test for hepatitis C virus (HCV). If you were born earlier or later and are at high risk for HCV infection, you may also need a blood test. |
| HIV testing | Get tested for HIV at least once. Discuss your risk with your doctor or nurse to determine if you need more frequent tests. |
| Lung cancer | If you are between ages 55 and 80, have smoked the equivalent of a pack of cigarettes a day for 30 years, and currently smoke or have quit within the past 15 years, you should have a low-dose CT scan annually. |
| Osteoporosis | Have a dual energy x-ray absorptiometry (DEXA) scan at least once after age 65. Talk to your doctor about repeat testing. |
| Pap smear | If you have a cervix, get a Pap test and human papillomavirus (HPV) test together every five years until age 65. Talk to your doctor about repeat testing after age 65. |
| Sexually transmitted diseases | Get tested for chlamydia, gonorrhea, and syphilis if you are at increased risk. |
| Tests at well-woman and preventive care visits | Insurance plans are required to cover a yearly well-woman visit for women under 65. Medicare covers a preventive care visit for women 65 or older. During these visits, you should be screened for high blood pressure, obesity, alcohol abuse, and depression. |

*Source: U.S. Preventive Services Task Force.*

## Table 4: Immunizations for women ages 50 or older

| IMMUNIZATION | RECOMMENDATION |
|---|---|
| Chickenpox (varicella) | You should get this vaccine once if you did not have chickenpox unless you have a weakened immune system. |
| Flu | You should get a flu shot every year. A high-dose version is available for people over 65. |
| Haemophilus flu (*Haemophilus influenzae* type b or Hib vaccine) | You should have this vaccination if your spleen has been removed or if you have a weakened immune system. Your doctor may recommend it if you have other risk factors or chronic conditions. |
| Hepatitis A | You should have this vaccination if you have chronic liver disease. Your doctor may recommend it if you have other chronic conditions. |
| Hepatitis B | You should have this vaccination if you have chronic liver disease, kidney disease, or HIV infection. Your doctor may recommend it if you have other risk factors or chronic conditions. |
| Meningitis (MenB as well as MenACWY or MSV4) | You should have this vaccination if your spleen has been removed. Your doctor may recommend it if you have other risk factors or chronic conditions. |
| Pneumonia | If you are 65 or older, you should get one dose of the PCV13 vaccine and at least one dose of the PPSV23 vaccine, depending on your age and health. |
| Shingles (varicella-zoster) | If you are 60 or older, you need a shingles vaccination, even if you have already had shingles. |
| Tetanus | You need at least one tetanus shot, included in the Tdap vaccine, followed by a booster every 10 years. |

*Source: CDC.*

years before serious consequences become apparent.

**Pay attention to your body.** Keep an eye on new spots and bumps, and note any changes in your regular patterns, be they in appetite, sleep, energy, bowel habits, or mood. It's easy to write off many changes as consequences of aging, but they could signal underlying disease.

**Be realistic.** No medical treatment, whether a knee replacement or a facelift, will restore you to your 20-year-old self. Accept a few minor aches and pains as a consequence of overexertion. If you have a chronic condition like fibromyalgia or irritable bowel syndrome, be prepared to try a number of therapies before finding the one, or the combination, that works best for you.

## 8 Stay connected

Women are living longer, and with aging comes the risk of isolation, as you retire and as your friends, partners, and relatives go into a steep decline or die. Society is more mobile today, so many of your friends and neighbors may also move away. This means that as you age, you need to work harder to maintain and bolster your local social connections in order to enhance your health into old age. Informal socializing with friends is of particular importance. Numerous studies have charted the positive influence of social networks on health later in life. For example, the Baltimore Longitudinal Study on Aging and the Georgia Cente-

narian Study have both found that older adults who remain socially active live longer and healthier lives than their solitary counterparts. The type of pursuit didn't matter. Activities ranged from bridge clubs to group travel to part-time jobs. Building connections in your local community is important, since studies show that trusted friends and neighbors make it more comfortable for you to walk and stay active in the neighborhood, get help from a neighbor, get help with chores, and share rides to keep up with health screenings.

## 9 Say no to stress

We all have stress in our lives. Whether it comes from a death in the family, the pain of arthritis, or a demanding job, the effects on the body are the same: The brain triggers a cascade of chemicals and hormones that speed heart rate, quicken breathing, increase blood pressure, and boost the amount of energy (in the form of blood sugar) supplied to muscles. Blood becomes "stickier" and more likely to clot, while the immune system releases inflammatory compounds. Intermittent episodes of stress are not harmful; in fact, you experience many of these symptoms during excitement and pleasure. However, chronic stress is a major contributor to a host of serious physical and psychological conditions.

Whatever sets your stress cycle in motion, having a personal escape plan can help you manage stressful

situations and even nip stress in the bud. To create a plan, make a list of the specific mental, emotional, and physical sensations that you feel when stressed. For example, do you get a stomachache, grind your teeth, raid the fridge, or have trouble thinking clearly? Whenever you notice your stress symptoms, take a moment—or two, or three— to relax. Here are some suggestions from Dr. Herbert Benson, president of the Benson-Henry Institute for Mind Body Medicine at Massachusetts General Hospital, depending on how much time you have:

**If you have one minute.** Place your hand just beneath your navel so you can feel the gentle rise and fall of your belly as you breathe. Breathe in slowly. Pause for a count of three. Exhale slowly. Pause for a count of three. Continue to breathe deeply for one minute, pausing for a count of three after each inhalation and exhalation.

**If you have two minutes.** Count down slowly from 10 to zero. With each number, take one complete breath, inhaling and exhaling. For example, breathe in deeply saying "10" to yourself. Breathe out slowly. On your next breath, say "nine," and so on. If you feel lightheaded, count down more slowly to space your breaths further apart. When you reach zero, you should feel more relaxed. If not, go through the exercise again.

**If you have three minutes.** While sitting down, take a break from whatever you're doing and check your body for tension. Relax your facial muscles and allow your jaw to fall open slightly. Let your shoulders drop. Let your arms fall to your sides. Allow your hands to loosen so that there are spaces between your fingers. Uncross your legs or ankles. Feel your thighs sink into your chair, letting your legs fall comfortably apart. Feel your shins and calves become heavier and your feet grow roots into the floor. Now breathe in slowly and breathe out slowly.

Dr. Benson offers two other simple tools for stress reduction: the worry box and the gratitude journal. The first is a repository for concerns that are beyond your power to influence—the safety of your children or grandchildren, the direction of the stock market, the heating of the planet. Write each worry on a slip of paper, put it in the box, and forget about it for at least a week. The second is a ritual—reflecting on the positive experiences and encounters of the day. Every night, jot down in a journal three good things that happened to you that day. Be specific. Don't write generalities, such as "I love my family," but concrete things that happened—a stunning sunset, a hug from your child, a compliment from a friend. Conjure up the scene in your mind and try to write about it in detail. If you do this every day, even after the worst of days, it will quickly become a habit for you to look for the all the things that are going right in your life, rather than fixating on what's going wrong. It will help you develop a new appreciation of your circumstances.

## ⑩ Shy away from supplements

People used to think that you could compensate for dietary deficiencies by popping a multivitamin every day. But the benefits of multivitamins remain uncertain. The Women's Health Initiative concluded that postmenopausal women who took multivitamins did not have a lower death rate than non-users of vitamins and were just as likely to develop cardiovascular disease or cancers of the lung, colon and rectum, breast, and endometrium. Other studies have similarly found little or no evidence of protection against cardiovascular disease or cancer from taking individual supplements such as vitamin E, vitamin C, beta carotene, or the popular B vitamin trio of $B_6$, $B_{12}$, and folic acid.

Research even suggests that excessive use of supplements may be harmful. A Cochrane Collaboration review found that low-risk participants in trials for a host of diseases who were given supplements of vitamin A, vitamin E, and beta carotene had a slightly higher death rate. And evidence has been mounting in recent years that people who consume the highest levels of calcium in the form of supplements may be more likely to have heart attacks or heart disease. Both observations, however, warrant further study.

Experts agree that the best way to get the nutrients we need is through food. No pill can make up for the fiber, antioxidants, and myriad other healthful compounds in fruits, vegetables, and legumes. It is likely that what counts is the synergistic interactions of these nutrients—which might also help explain why trials of single nutrients often don't pan out.

To be sure, there may be supplements worth considering. Calcium and vitamin D are essential for preserving bone density, but the long-standing recommendation of 1,200 mg of calcium for women over 50 has been called into question as mounting evidence indicates that a calcium intake that high has little effect on bone density and may increase the risk of kidney stones. Many experts consider a daily intake of 500 to 700 mg—a level recommended by the World Health Organization—adequate. Still, many women fall short on vitamin D. The government recommends 600 IU a day for women ages 51 to 70; 800 IU for women over age 71. But many health experts now recommend getting 1,000 IU, which is harder to do without taking supplements. And if you are vegan or vegetarian, you may need to take vitamin $B_{12}$, an essential vitamin for the nerves, which is found in animal-based foods. Consult your doctor about what supplements may be right for you. ◆

# Minimizing potentially disabling disorders

Although the disorders in this chapter—both physical and psychological—might not rob your life of years, they can rob your years of life. Some, like osteoporosis, may sideline you with a hip or spinal fracture, while others, like depression, may make it hard to get out of bed. Arthritis may impair your ability to do simple tasks; so may anxiety. Some of these ailments are preventable; some are curable; all are treatable.

## Osteoporosis

If you're over 50, the odds that you'll experience a major fracture because of osteoporosis at some point in your life are one in two—much higher than the one-in-six risk faced by men. This disorder weakens bones, leaving them vulnerable to breaking even without a serious fall or other trauma. Postmenopausal women are twice as likely as men the same age to have an osteoporotic fracture, because they have smaller bones to begin with and because bone loss is accelerated by the decline in estrogen at menopause. And because women are living longer than ever, osteoporosis is a significant cause of disability later in life.

Osteoporosis increases the risk of fractures in every bone of the body. However, two types of osteoporotic fractures—in the spine and hip—can be particularly disabling.

In the spine, compression fractures can cause vertebrae to collapse. Multiple spinal compression fractures in a woman can lead to a medical condition called dorsal kyphosis, or "dowager's hump" (see Figure 6, at right). The collapsed vertebrae may cause a downward curve in the top section of the spine and a loss in height between the shoulder and hip. As the length of the torso shrinks, the abdominal organs are crowded and pushed forward, leading to a host of discomforts, including breathing difficulties, digestive disorders, constipation, and urinary incontinence.

Moreover, the changes can throw off your balance, making it more difficult to get around.

Hip fractures usually involve cracks in the head of the femur, or thighbone. Because these injuries usually occur later in life, the road to recovery can be difficult. Repair usually involves hip replacement and many weeks of recovery and rehabilitation treatments.

### Preventing osteoporosis

While it's true that all people lose bone as they age, osteoporosis is not inevitable; there are still many things you can do to hold on to the bone you have and perhaps even replace some lost bone.

**Quit smoking.** Tobacco use has been linked to lower bone density, and it's clear that smoking increases fracture risk. But the exact reasons are hard to pin down, as smokers also tend to be thin, drink alcohol, have poor diets, and enter menopause earlier, all of which increase the risk of osteoporosis.

---

**Figure 6: Bent backs**

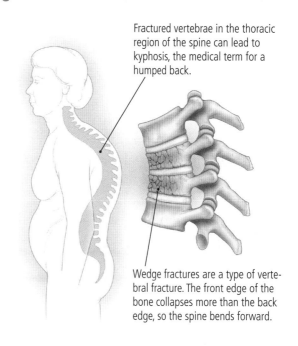

Fractured vertebrae in the thoracic region of the spine can lead to kyphosis, the medical term for a humped back.

Wedge fractures are a type of vertebral fracture. The front edge of the bone collapses more than the back edge, so the spine bends forward.

**Eat a balanced diet.** If you don't supply your body with the calcium it needs, it will respond by raiding calcium stores in your bones. You can find calcium in vegetables such as leafy greens, as well as low-fat dairy and fortified foods. Vitamin D, which helps your body absorb calcium, is harder to obtain through your diet, but you can find it in egg yolks, saltwater fish, and liver. Aim for a total calcium intake of 500 mg to 800 mg daily, mostly through foods. The National Osteoporosis Foundation currently recommends 800 to 1,000 international units (IU) of vitamin D per day for bone health (which is higher than the government's recommendation for overall health; see "Shy away from supplements," page 28), but some experts think that even 1,000 IU daily isn't enough. In addition, stick to these daily limits:

- No more than three cups of coffee or the equivalent. It seems that high levels of caffeine increase calcium excretion in the kidneys. In an observational study of 66,000 women, those consuming four or more cups of coffee daily had a 4% lower average bone density in the spine and a 2% lower density at the hip than women who drank only one cup a day.

- No more than 0.8 grams of protein per kilogram of your weight (about 45 grams for a 125-pound woman). High levels of protein are thought to increase calcium excretion through the kidneys. In response, calcium may be released from bones to restore calcium balance in the blood.

- No more than 700 micrograms (2,300 IU) of vitamin A. There is some evidence that higher amounts of vitamin A stimulate the production of osteoclasts, the cells that break down bone.

**Do weight-bearing exercise.** Any exercise that involves working against gravity, such as running, walking, weight lifting, or stair climbing, can potentially build bone. Because activities like swimming and bicycling aren't weight-bearing, they don't help strengthen bones. Aim to get at least 30 minutes of weight-bearing exercise a day. Exercise also increases muscle mass, which can help protect bones from injury, and it improves strength, agility, and flexibility, thus decreasing susceptibility to falls.

**Avoid excess alcohol.** Excess alcohol has many adverse effects on bone. It interferes with calcium

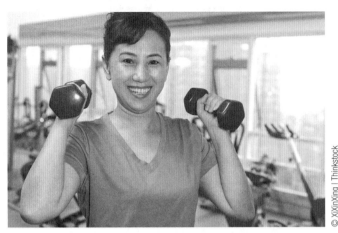

Weight-bearing exercise helps to keep your bones strong. But the term "weight-bearing" is often misunderstood. While it includes classic strength training, it also includes anything that involves working against gravity, such as running.

balance and alters bone-building hormones, including estrogen and cortisol. And because drinking too much can make you unsteady on your feet, you're more likely to fall and break a bone. Try to limit daily consumption to one drink of wine, beer, or spirits (see Figure 5, page 24).

**Get a bone density screening.** As menopause recedes into the rear-view mirror, it's even more important to track your bone density. The World Health Organization (WHO) has developed criteria for diagnosing osteoporosis based on a measurement of bone mineral density called a T-score. These scores are most frequently determined by dual energy x-ray absorptiometry (DEXA). A T-score of –2.5 or lower marks the threshold for osteoporosis.

Most experts recommend DEXA screening for all women ages 65 and over. Other women at high risk of bone loss should also be screened—namely, postmenopausal women ages 45 to 64 who weigh 132 pounds or less, and women ages 55 to 64 who weigh 154 or less and are not taking estrogen.

In 2008, a WHO task force also introduced FRAX, a risk-assessment tool that incorporates a number of risk factors besides bone density. The tool, which is available online (www.shef.ac.uk/FRAX), provides an estimate of the likelihood that you will fracture a hip or have another major fracture in the next 10 years. Using FRAX, the National Osteoporosis Foundation issued guidelines suggesting that clinicians consider treatment with an FDA-approved drug for women who meet any of the following criteria:

- a history of hip or spine fracture
- a T-score of less than –2.5 at the hip or spine
- a T-score of –1.0 to –2.5 at the hip or spine (indicating osteopenia, which is low bone mass short of osteoporosis) together with a 10-year, FRAX-estimated risk of more than 20% for any major osteoporosis-related fracture or more than 3% for hip fracture.

If you fall into one of those categories, exercise and a diet rich in calcium and vitamin D alone won't provide sufficient bone protection. You may also need to take a bone-building medication. Many women worry about possible side effects from osteoporosis drugs, including fractures in the upper thighbone. Although these fractures are very rare, an expert task force concluded that they were indeed a possible consequence of long-term (five years or more) use of drugs known as bisphosphonates, including as alendronate (Fosamax), risedronate (Actonel), and ibandronate (Boniva). As a result, the FDA issued a warning in 2010, and clinicians now often recommend that women who've used these medications for a while take a "drug holiday," stopping the drug for at least a while. If you and your doctor do decide that you should stop, be sure to have your bone density tested after a year or two. If it has declined significantly, you can always resume medication. If you're taking bisphosphonates, have the need for continued therapy re-evaluated on a periodic basis.

# Osteoarthritis

Osteoarthritis, the most common type of arthritis, is also called a degenerative disease because it results from the deterioration of the bones and cartilage that make up the joints. From ages 40 to 70, osteoarthritis is more common in women than men. Women more often have osteoarthritis in the hands and knees and are 10 times more likely to develop Heberden's nodes—hard, bony growths that form on the joint nearest the fingertip.

Osteoarthritis can result from genetics and also from trauma or repeated stress. In the knees, osteoarthritis may be the result of years of skiing, tennis, or another sport that torques the knee joints. Women with this problem may find it increasingly difficult to walk, climb stairs, or get up from a chair.

Osteoarthritis of the hand often starts with stiffness and soreness of the joint at the base of the thumb (see Figure 7, below), particularly in the morning. Some people with osteoarthritis of the hand may find that with age, their hands thicken and become stiff. Stiffness is gradually followed by pain or instability. In other people, pain and stiffness may subside over time, leaving only enlarged joints as reminders.

## Living with arthritis

Arthritis can be disruptive and disconcerting. The pain and stiffness can make it difficult to perform the daily tasks most people take for granted. Simple activities like dressing yourself or cooking dinner can become a major effort. The following strategies and therapies can make coping with arthritis a little easier.

**Regular exercise.** It may be counterintuitive, but physical activity not only helps maintain joint function, but also relieves stiffness and decreases pain and fatigue. Exercise can also help to increase range of motion, strengthen muscles, and build endurance.

## Figure 7: Osteoarthritis of the hand

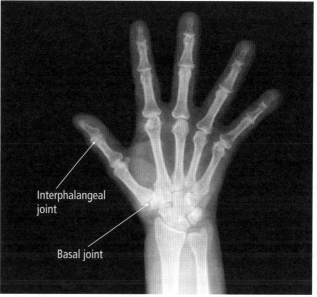

Reprinted with permission from Barry P. Simmons, M.D.

Osteoarthritis is visible in the two joints of the thumb where the normal joint space is narrowed, causing restricted movement and discomfort.

As little as an hour to two hours of moderate physical activity each week should start to produce results. Work with your clinician or physical therapist to develop your own exercise routine.

**Achieving and maintaining a normal body weight.** Bearing excess weight results in more stress on joints and more pain.

**Assistive devices.** A wide variety of splints are available by prescription and over the counter for hands and fingers, wrists, elbows, knees, and ankles. These may help to ease pain and increase mobility. Using a cane can relieve pressure on hips and knees substantially. An increasing array of helpful gadgets, from jar openers to dusters to garden pruners, are also available online and at home and hardware stores.

**Acupuncture.** A meta-analysis of 24 studies found that acupuncture significantly improved pain in people with hip or knee osteoarthritis. If you are considering acupuncture, find a licensed practitioner. Keep in mind that acupuncture isn't covered by Medicare and may not be covered by your insurer either.

**Heat therapy.** A warm shower or bath can work wonders anytime, especially before and after exercising. Hot packs and moist or dry heating pads, or even a folded towel warmed in the oven or microwave, can offer instant relief.

**Cooling.** Gel-filled cold packs, coolant sprays, ice chips in a plastic bag, and packages of frozen peas can soothe hot, painful joints. To avoid disrupting circulation to the joint, don't leave them on longer than 20 minutes.

## Drug treatment for osteoarthritis

Medication works best with other pain relief strategies, such as exercising to build your muscles and protect your joints from injury. Options include the following:

**Topical pain relievers.** Applied to the skin, these offer one alternative for mild pain relief. Creams containing salicylate (Aspercreme, Bengay) and others containing capsaicin (Capsaicin, Zostrix) are available over the counter.

**Oral drugs.** Doctors often recommend acetaminophen (Tylenol) first because it's effective for mild pain and easy on the stomach. However, nonsteroidal anti-inflammatory drugs (NSAIDs) are generally considered more effective than acetaminophen in treating osteoarthritis because they reduce inflammation as well as pain. The arsenal of NSAIDs includes over-the-counter medications such as aspirin, ibuprofen (Advil, Motrin), and naproxen (Aleve), as well as the prescription drugs diclofenac (Voltaren), indomethacin (Indocin), meloxicam (Mobic), and nabumetone (Relafen). Because NSAIDs, particularly aspirin and indomethacin, inhibit the enzyme that protects the stomach lining and interfere with blood clotting, they increase the risks of bleeding and gastric ulcers. Some of the prescription NSAIDs, particularly nabumetone, meloxicam, and diclofenac, seem to be relatively gentler on the digestive system. Some formulations, such as Arthrotec (diclofenac and misoprostol) or Prevacid NapraPAC (lansoprazole and naproxen), combine an NSAID with a medication that protects the stomach.

**Glucosamine and chondroitin.** Glucosamine and chondroitin are chemical components of cartilage, and in theory, supplements containing synthetic versions of these substances might help stop joint destruction and ease arthritis pain. However, the results of clinical trials have been inconclusive. The largest study, the 1,500-person NIH-sponsored Glucosamine/Chondroitin Arthritis Intervention Trial (GAIT), found that the supplements, either alone or in combination, were no more effective than a dummy pill, or placebo, in slowing the progression of arthritis of the knee or relieving knee pain. However, they seemed to be more effective than the placebo in providing relief for the 22% of participants who had moderate to severe pain. The supplements' side effects are minimal, but they may increase bleeding in people who take warfarin (Coumadin). As always, if you choose to take these or any other alternative preparations, be sure to inform your physician.

**Injections.** Corticosteroid injections into the joint can relieve inflammation quickly, but usually only for a short time. They are recommended no more than two to three times a year, and only when absolutely necessary, because they may increase the risk of infection and can further damage the joints. Another alternative, hyaluronate (Hyalgan, Synvisc), is a synthetic version of a natural lubricant in the joint. It can be injected directly into the knee at weekly intervals for three to five weeks. However, the modest benefits experienced by some people may not be worth the discomfort of the injections.

### Surgery for osteoarthritis

Surgical options are usually recommended when drug therapies and other strategies are no longer effective, but before mobility is seriously limited.

**Arthroscopy.** Usually reserved for the knees, arthroscopy is considered minor surgery because the incisions are small and the procedure generally does not require an overnight stay in the hospital. An arthroscope (an instrument with a tiny light and a camera) and a variety of miniaturized surgical instruments are inserted into the joint through different small incisions. If there is torn cartilage to repair or debris to remove, the procedure can result in mild to moderate improvement that may last several months or perhaps a few years. It may be helpful if other treatments have failed, but recent studies have questioned its usefulness for most cases of osteoarthritis.

**Joint reconstruction or replacement.** Surgery can be used to correct joint deformity, to reconstruct a joint, or to completely replace a diseased joint with a prosthetic device. Long-term data from knee and hip replacements indicate that a prosthetic joint will last an average of 10 to 15 years and should relieve your pain substantially. Moreover, thanks to improved materials, newer prostheses may last even longer. If you're considering hip or knee replacement, you should be committed to participating in weeks of physical therapy after surgery.

**Alternatives to joint replacement.** While joint replacement is considered the definitive treatment for a badly damaged knee or hip, it is generally considered a last resort and is not right for everyone. Other options include the following:

- **Realignment.** Surgery can be performed to realign bones that are no longer correctly lined up as a result of osteoarthritis.
- **Fusion.** Another possibility involves permanently fusing two bones at the affected joint. This is an option when arthritis occurs in parts of the body such as the wrist, ankle, and small joints of the fingers and toes, where joint replacement is less reliable and rarely performed.
- **Hip resurfacing.** Instead of removing the head of the femur and replacing it with an artificial ball, the surgeon reshapes the head and caps it with a cobalt-chromium prosthetic that fits into an artificial metal lining in the socket. Resurfacing uses a bigger ball than hip replacement does, which some surgeons say makes dislocation less likely and gives the joint the ability handle greater stress.

# Foot problems

Simply getting older puts women at risk for foot problems. With age, the fatty pads on the bottoms of your feet become thinner and less able to absorb shock. Your feet get longer and wider because of age-related stretching of ligaments and tendons. Wearing shoes with high heels and narrow toes is also a major contributor to pain. As a result, women have four times as many foot problems as men and account for 90% of surgical procedures for common foot ailments. The following are some of the most frequent disorders.

### Bunions

A bunion is a bump of bone or tissue that forms at the big toe joint—or, less frequently, at the joint of the little toe. It can rub against the inside of a shoe, causing inflammation of the bursa (the fluid-filled sac surrounding the metatarsal joint) and considerable pain.

**Conservative treatment.** Warm soaks or ice packs, along with NSAIDs, should relieve pain. When you're on the go, protect the bunion with a moleskin pad or a semisoft orthotic insert placed in your shoe. Wearing sneakers, running shoes, or shoes with roomy toes is essential.

**Surgery.** A bunionectomy, sometimes accompanied by cutting and repositioning foot bones, is usually successful. Recovery may take six months and require wearing a cast or special shoes.

### Plantar fasciitis

If you have pain at the bottom of your foot just in front of the heel, you may have inflammation of the plantar fascia, a band of ligaments and tendons that stretches from the heel bone to the bones of the toes. The fascia forms the arch of the foot and is a shock absorber for the body. Plantar fasciitis can result from an uneven stride, poorly designed shoes, or chronic overuse during high-impact exercise.

**Conservative treatment.** The best therapy for plantar fasciitis is rest and cushioning the heel, either by wearing a good walking or running shoe or by using orthotics. Taking NSAIDs will reduce inflammation. After the pain has begun to subside, you should stretch the foot gently through low-impact exercise such as swimming and bicycling.

**Aggressive treatment.** If your pain is severe and unremitting, your doctor may suggest steroid injections. Orthotripsy, an outpatient procedure in which shock waves are directed at the affected heel, may also be effective. Surgery to release the fascia is a last resort.

### Hammertoes

This deformity of the joints causes toes to bend up and curl under like a claw. Sometimes it's caused by heredity, arthritis, or a too-tight tendon, but more often it's the consequence of ill-fitting shoes. A narrow shoe with a tight toe box aggravates the condition, forcing the toe to bump up against the upper part of the shoe.

**Conservative treatment.** As long as the hammertoe is flexible, roomier shoes and a toe pad to keep the toe from rubbing on the shoe should relieve some of the pain. Exercises, splints, and orthotics will help position the toe more comfortably.

**Surgery.** If the hammertoe has become stiff, it's harder to treat and may require an in-office procedure under local anesthesia to remove a small piece of bone so that the toe can return to a normal position. Recovery takes one to four weeks and usually requires wearing a splint and surgical shoe.

### Neuroma

Nerve irritation can produce a burning sensation or numbness in the foot and may be responsible for the development of a painful lump or thickening of tissue. In women, neuroma is due mostly to wearing narrow shoes with high heels or a constricting vamp (the section of shoe upper that covers the front of the foot). Arthritis and repetitive stress can also cause the condition.

**Conservative treatment.** Neuromas can be treated with massage and by wearing roomier shoes fitted with protective pads or orthotics. Cortisone injections can also relieve pain.

**Surgery.** A neurectomy (surgical removal of all or part of the nerve) should relieve the pain, but it may also leave a portion of the toes without feeling. Recovery from a neurectomy usually takes two to three months.

## Depression

One of the most prevalent medical conditions in the United States, depression affects one in four women at some point. Scientists and clinicians have come to speak of the "depressive illnesses," a term encompassing major depression, persistent depressive disorder (formerly known as dysthymia), bipolar disorder, and seasonal affective disorder (SAD; see "Four common patterns of depression," page 35). While every person's experience of depression is unique, any of these symptoms may occur:

- a persistent sad or empty mood
- loss of interest or pleasure in formerly enjoyable activities
- fatigue or lack of energy
- sleep disruptions
- eating disturbances
- difficulty concentrating, remembering, or making decisions
- feelings of guilt, worthlessness, or helplessness
- thoughts of death or suicide
- irritability
- inappropriate or excessive crying
- aches and pains
- other symptoms that do not respond to treatment.

Many factors, both biological and experiential, contribute to depression. Moods arise in and are regulated by the brain. The systems we have in place to manage mood may break down in several ways. A woman's genetic endowment may make her vulnerable. There may be subtle problems in the structure of nerve cells or the way that nerve cells convey signals to one another. Cells make up circuits and brain regions, all of which must communicate properly. The

## Four common patterns of depression

**1** **Major depression.** This is the classic form of depression, where a dark mood is all-consuming, or one loses interest in activities, even ones that are usually pleasurable. Classic symptoms of depression include trouble sleeping, changes in appetite or weight, loss of energy, and feeling worthless. Thoughts of death or suicide may occur. Major depression is more common in women than men and can occur at any age. An episode may be precipitated by a loss, but it can also crop up without warning, unrelated to life events. In this state of mind, it may be difficult to find the energy to seek treatment, but treatment is usually necessary to get relief.

**2** **Persistent depressive disorder.** Formerly called "dysthymia," this term refers to low mood that is long-lasting but may not reach the intensity of major depression. Many people with this are able to function day to day, but feel low or joyless much of the time. They may come to believe that it is normal to feel blue. Some depressive symptoms, such as appetite and sleep changes, low energy, low self-esteem, or hopelessness, are usually part of the picture. For a diagnosis, these symptoms must have persisted at least for two years, but there is no need to wait a specific length of time to get help. Treatment can provide effective relief.

**3** **Bipolar disorder.** People with bipolar disorder—once known as manic-depressive disease—have episodes of depression. But they also go through periods of unusually high energy or activity. The most florid episodes are called "mania." Manic symptoms look like the opposite of depression symptoms: grandiose ideas, unrealistically high self-esteem, decreased need for sleep, thoughts and activity at higher speed, and ramped-up pursuit of pleasure including sex sprees, overspending, and risk taking. Being manic can feel great, but it doesn't last long and can lead to self-destructive behavior. Pharmacological treatments for bipolar disorder are different from other depressive disorders, but can be very effective at stabilizing a person's mood.

**4** **Seasonal affective disorder (SAD).** This form of depression emerges as days get shorter in the fall and winter. The mood change may result from alterations in the body's natural daily rhythms, in the eyes' sensitivity to light, or in how chemical messengers like serotonin and melatonin function. The leading treatment is light therapy, which involves daily sessions sitting close to an especially intense light source. The usual treatments for depression, such as psychotherapy and medication, are also acceptable.

brain also changes in response to the environment—relationships with loved ones, stressful life events, early experiences with caregivers, or exposures to medications, to name a few. Scientists are only beginning to understand all of these complicated relationships.

Together with the acknowledgment of this complexity has come the recognition that depression is not a sign of personal weakness; rather, it is a serious medical condition requiring professional treatment. Risk factors for depression include the following:

- a family history of depression, particularly in first-degree relatives
- a parent who has committed suicide
- a personal history of substance abuse or an eating disorder, or a family history of such disorders
- unresolved grief over a major life loss
- unresolved anger.

### Why women get depressed

Although there is general agreement that numerous factors contribute to a higher rate of depression in women, the nature of those factors is a subject of ongoing debate. The commonly acknowledged ones include emotional "hardwiring," developmental experiences, and social conditioning.

These factors are interrelated. Women are considered to be more responsive to signals from others and more reliant on external feedback for their sense of self. Women are also more likely than men to repress anger or aggression or to turn those feelings on themselves, rather than to vent them appropriately. Moreover, society expects the "good" woman to subordinate her needs to those of others. All these tendencies contribute to a loss of self-esteem—a central feature of depression.

The stage for depression during adulthood may be set quite early in life. As girls, many older women were taught that reticence and modesty were traits to be cultivated, and they learned to defer to boys in the classroom and in social situations. Being habitually relegated to the background can erode one's sense of self-worth. The stresses of adolescence—including the struggle for independence, the dawning awareness of one's sexuality, increased freedom to make one's own decisions, hormonal changes, and, often, a negative body image—can also play a role.

Although it was once widely believed that depression was a common consequence of menopause, a number of population-based studies have failed to demonstrate an increase in the rate of depression at midlife. In fact, it can work either way. When the end of fertility comes at the same time that one's children are entering adolescence or leaving home, some women experience a sense of loss; in contrast, many others find the release from the possibility of pregnancy to be a liberating experience.

However, more women than men become depressed late in life, when women often have more risk factors for depression, such as social isolation and bereavement.

## Identifying depression

It's important to note that depression is often associated with certain medical conditions. It can be precipitated by a stroke, heart attack, or cancer, or by the use of some medications. Because depression can be responsible for memory loss or for difficulty in reasoning, it is often mistakenly identified in older women as dementia or Alzheimer's disease. It can also coexist with another mental illness. In such cases, the clinician usually identifies one disorder as the "primary" condition and treats it first.

If you suspect that you have one of the depressive disorders, don't wait for your clinician to detect your condition. Ask for a diagnostic evaluation. Because depression is a mind-body disorder, both a general physical and a psychiatric evaluation are recommended. The physical can identify or rule out other causes, such as hypothyroidism, and may help to determine your fitness to undergo treatment for depression. The psychiatric evaluation can help to establish the problem's intensity and to detect any other emotional disorders that may be present.

## Treating depression

For most people, the immediate goal is to feel and function better as quickly as possible. In general, the milder the disorder, the more numerous the options for treating it. The two most common approaches are antidepressant medications and psychotherapy. Studies have indicated that either of these approaches or a combination of both can be effective for treating depression.

**Drug treatment.** There are many factors to consider when selecting an antidepressant. Because chemistry is an important determinant of anyone's response to antidepressants, some drugs will be more effective than others for any given person. Moreover, each antidepressant is associated with a slightly different set of side effects—for example, loss of libido, constipation, sleep disturbances, or weight gain—which can influence your choice. While your clinician should have an idea of the drugs that are likely to be effective for you, you should let him or her know which side effects you consider the most or least tolerable.

Because several weeks of treatment may be necessary for an antidepressant to become fully effective, it is important not to give up on a drug too soon. Your clinician should be able to judge when you have given a medication an adequate trial. It is often necessary to try a few antidepressants before finding a drug that effectively relieves symptoms and whose side effects are tolerable. As a general rule, drugs alone are most successful when the depression is not exacerbated by an ongoing stressful situation.

**Psychotherapy.** Talk therapy is most effective in the hands of a skilled professional who is also a good fit with the person. Therapy can provide insight into the specific factors that precipitated the depression; guidance in changing thoughts, feelings, and behaviors that may fuel the disorder; and aid in dealing with the condition's effects on work and relationships. Moreover, it helps to have the support of a therapist when living with the side effects of antidepressants and the potential frustration of trying several medications unsuccessfully.

However, even the most gifted therapist is not a magician who can dispel gloom immediately. Several weeks may elapse before the sessions produce a noticeable change in mood. It's important to give the process a chance, even though you may feel that you are accomplishing little at first.

**Electroconvulsive therapy (ECT).** This procedure, in which controlled seizures are induced under general anesthesia to alter brain chemistry, is usually reserved for people with severe depression for whom antidepressants have been ineffective or who are considered to be in danger of suicide. Because it is relatively fast-acting, ECT's major role is in "jump-starting" treatment. It often produces a loss of recent memory, which usually resolves over time.

**Light therapy.** Controlled exposure to full-spectrum light has helped some people with SAD. Early studies indicate that it may have a role in treating other types of depression as well.

# Anxiety

Nearly two-thirds of the estimated 57 million adults with anxiety disorders are women. What these disorders have in common is unwarranted fear or distress that interferes with daily life (see Table 5, below).

Anxiety is a reaction to stress that has both psychological and physical features. The feeling is thought to arise in the amygdala, a brain region that governs many intense emotional responses. As neurotransmitters carry the impulse to the sympathetic nervous system, heart and breathing rates increase, muscles tense, and blood flow is diverted from the abdominal organs to the brain.

Some degree of anxiety is normal and even necessary. In the short term, it prepares us to confront a crisis by putting the body on alert and prompting us to take extra precautions. But its physical effects can be counterproductive, causing lightheadedness, nausea, diarrhea, and frequent urination. And when anxiety persists, it can not only interfere with our daily lives but also undermine our physical health. Evidence suggests that people with anxiety disorders are at greater risk for developing a number of chronic medical conditions. They may also have more severe symptoms, and women with anxiety have a greater risk of death when they become ill.

Research on the physiology of anxiety-related illness is still young, but there's growing evidence of mutual influence between emotions and physical functioning. Yet anxiety often goes unidentified as a source of other disorders, such as substance abuse or physical addiction, that can result from attempts to quell feelings of anxiety.

Anxiety plays a role in somatoform disorders—mental disorders that are characterized by physical symptoms such as pain, nausea, weakness, or dizziness that have no apparent physical cause. It has also been implicated in several chronic physical illnesses, including heart disease, chronic respiratory disorders, and gastrointestinal conditions. When people with these disorders have untreated anxiety, the disease itself is more difficult to treat, their physical symptoms often worsen, and in some cases they die sooner.

## Table 5: Anxiety disorders and their symptoms

| DISORDER | SYMPTOMS |
|---|---|
| Generalized anxiety disorder | Exaggerated worry about health, safety, money, and other aspects of daily life that lasts six months or more. Often accompanied by muscle pain, fatigue, headaches, nausea, breathlessness, and insomnia. |
| Obsessive-compulsive disorder (OCD) | Obsessive thoughts, such as an irrational fear of contamination, accompanied by compulsive acts, such as repetitive hand washing, that are undertaken to alleviate the anxiety generated by the thoughts. |
| Panic disorder | Recurrent episodes of unprovoked feelings of terror or impending doom, accompanied by rapid heartbeat, sweating, dizziness, or weakness. |
| Phobias | Irrational fear of specific things or situations, such as spiders (arachnophobia), being in crowds (agoraphobia), or being in enclosed spaces (claustrophobia). |
| Post-traumatic stress disorder (PTSD) | Reliving an intense physical or emotional threat or injury (for example, childhood abuse, combat, or an earthquake) in vivid dreams, flashbacks, or tormented memories. Other symptoms include difficulty sleeping or concentrating, angry outbursts, emotional withdrawal, and a heightened startle response. |
| Social anxiety disorder (social phobia) | Overwhelming self-consciousness in ordinary social encounters, heightened by a sense of being watched and judged by others and a fear of embarrassment. |

## Treating anxiety

When anxiety is related to a medical condition or to substance use, treatment focuses on the underlying causes. Otherwise, there are three primary approaches to treatment:

**Cognitive behavioral therapy.** The cognitive component helps people identify and avoid thoughts that generate anxiety, and the behavioral part helps them learn how to react differently to anxiety-provoking situations. The specifics of the treatment depend on the type of anxiety. For example, people with generalized anxiety disorder or panic disorder may be asked to examine their lives for habits and patterns that foster a sense of dread, and may also be taught relaxation techniques to diminish anxiety. People with obsessive-compulsive disorder characterized by excessive washing may be asked to dirty their hands and wait with a therapist for increasingly longer intervals before cleaning up.

**Psychodynamic psychotherapy.** Anxiety is often triggered by a deep-seated emotional conflict or a traumatic experience that can sometimes be explored and resolved through psychotherapy. In the first randomized controlled clinical trial comparing relaxation therapy to psychodynamic psychotherapy (focused talk therapy), clinician-researchers at Columbia University in New York found that people with panic disorder treated with psychodynamic therapy had significantly fewer symptoms and functioned better socially than those who underwent relaxation therapy. Nearly three-quarters of the psychotherapy group responded to treatment, compared with only 39% of the relaxation therapy group.

**Drug therapy.** Medications alone are less effective than psychotherapy over the long term; they may also have unpleasant side effects and interact with other medications. Still, they can be helpful when used in combination with psychotherapy. The most commonly used types of drugs include anti-anxiety medications, which act quickly but become less effective as tolerance builds; antidepressants, which may take longer to become effective but can be used for longer periods; and beta blockers, which reduce the physical response of anxiety by slowing heart rate and lowering blood pressure.

# Underactive thyroid

Midlife can bring subtle changes in skin, hair, energy, weight, and even mental outlook. Before writing these off as side effects of aging, it's a good idea to make sure they're not the result of an underactive thyroid.

This tiny butterfly-shaped gland influences virtually every organ system in the body. The hormones it secretes into the bloodstream play a vital role in regulating metabolism, the rate at which our bodies convert food and oxygen to energy. Low thyroid hormone production, or hypothyroidism, causes a range of symptoms—fatigue, constipation, dry skin, brittle nails, aches and pains, and feeling down—that you might easily attribute to other health problems.

Untreated hypothyroidism can increase your risk for high cholesterol, high blood pressure, and heart disease. But it is easily diagnosed with a blood test and treated with a pill. That's why it's important to keep an eye out for the symptoms and have your thyroid function checked.

## Symptoms of underactive thyroid

The symptoms of hypothyroidism can differ from person to person. In some women, the onset is so gradual that it's hardly noticeable; in others, symptoms come on abruptly over the course of a few weeks or months. In general, the lower thyroid hormone levels are, the more pronounced and severe the following symptoms will be:

**Fatigue.** Low thyroid function can result in less energy.

**Cold intolerance.** Slowed-down cells burn less energy, so the body produces less heat. You may feel chilly even when others around you are comfortable.

**Appetite loss, weight gain.** Although this seems contradictory, you may eat less and gain weight. The lower your energy requirements, the fewer calories you need, so your appetite declines. At the same time, you may gain a few pounds because your body converts fewer calories into energy, leaving more to be stored as fat.

**Cardiovascular effects.** Low levels of thyroid hormone can lead to high blood pressure as well as elevated levels of total and LDL cholesterol. The heart's pumping ability may fall, reducing blood flow to the skin, kidneys, brain, and other vital tissues, and increasing the risk of heart failure, especially in older women.

**Mental effects.** Hypothyroidism and depression share many of the same symptoms, including difficulty concentrating, memory problems, and loss of interest in things that are normally important to you. They call for different treatments, so proper diagnosis is important.

**Other signs and symptoms.** Hypothyroidism can act as a dimmer switch on nearly every bodily function. Digestive processes become sluggish, causing constipation. Speech and movement may slow. Muscle aches and pain around the joints, including carpal tunnel syndrome, are common. Skin, hair, and nails may become dry and thin.

If you have any of these symptoms, see your clinician for a physical exam. You'll be checked for physical signs of hypothyroidism, and you may have blood tests for levels of thyroid-stimulating hormone (TSH) as well as the thyroid hormone thyroxine (T4).

## Treating underactive thyroid

Hypothyroidism is usually treated with a daily dose of synthetic T4 (levothyroxine sodium), taken in pill form. Levothyroxine works exactly like your body's natural thyroid hormone. It's available in the generic form and under such brand names as Unithroid, Levothroid, Levoxyl, and Synthroid. Some people also require a small dose of synthetic T3 (Cytomel). The goal of drug treatment is to lower your TSH to about the midpoint of normal range and maintain it at that level. Typically, you'll start with a relatively low dose and have your TSH checked six to eight weeks later. If necessary, your physician will adjust the dose, repeating this process until your TSH is in the normal range. Once the right dose is established, your TSH and possibly T4 levels will be checked once or twice a year. Most people who take enough synthetic T4 to normalize TSH levels find that their symptoms disappear.

# Incontinence

The unintended loss of urine or feces can make it difficult to maintain good hygiene and carry on ordinary life. Besides disrupting daily activities and nighttime sleep, incontinence can also chip away at your health. If you have stopped exercising for fear of leakage, for example, you are giving up one of the most effective ways of maintaining health. If you're getting up several times a night to go to the bathroom, you're risking not only sleep deprivation but injury from falls. Older women who frequently must rush to the bathroom are 26% more likely to fall and 34% more likely to break a bone. The good news is that treatments are becoming better and easier. For example, new medicines for urinary incontinence are more effective, and most procedures for urinary incontinence can be done with minimally invasive techniques that require less time for recovery.

## Treating urinary incontinence

Urinary incontinence typically takes the form of stress incontinence or urge incontinence. Stress incontinence refers to urine leaking during exercise, sneezing, or coughing. It is often due to weakening of the pelvic floor muscles or urinary sphincter—the muscle that controls the opening of the bladder. Urge incontinence is caused by a bladder that contracts suddenly, often before it is full (a condition also known as overactive bladder). People with urge incontinence frequently experience a sudden and overwhelming urge to void and may leak urine if they can't get to a bathroom in time. Some women may have both stress and urge incontinence. Several approaches have been successful in relieving urge incontinence, stress incontinence, or both.

**Bladder control training.** Women with urge incontinence practice consciously suppressing the urge to urinate for progressively longer intervals.

**Fluid management.** This approach is based on minimizing alcohol, caffeine, and carbonated beverages; restricting daily fluids to less than 64 ounces daily; and drinking slowly and no more than 8 ounces at a time.

**Pelvic muscle strengthening.** Exercising the pelvic muscles by contracting them and releasing them (as though grasping a tampon) can be performed by doing Kegel exercises, or passively, with either electrical stimulation or pulsed magnetic fields. Biofeedback training may help you to locate and contract the muscles.

**Weight loss.** Studies have shown that weight loss helps alleviate symptoms, although researchers are not sure why. It may reduce abdominal pressure on the bladder.

**Medication.** Vaginal estrogen can used to help relieve all types of urinary incontinence if vaginal atrophy is present. There are currently no FDA-approved medications for stress incontinence. A class of drugs called antimuscarinics, which work by blocking nerve impulses to the bladder, can help with urge incontinence. A common side effect is a dry mouth.

**Pessaries.** A pessary is a device made of silicone that comes in a variety of shapes and sizes and is fitted into the vagina. Left in place there, the pessary compresses the urethra against the upper rear portion of the pubic bone, which can help prevent urinary leakage.

**Botox.** Injections of Botox are FDA-approved for treating overactive bladder when oral medications to inhibit bladder contractions can't be taken or are ineffective.

**Electrical stimulation.** Two treatment options for urge incontinence use nerve stimulation to control bladder contractions. One approach, called percutaneous tibial nerve stimulation (PTNS), involves using a device to send mild electrical pulses to the tibial nerve, just under the skin near the ankle. These pulses travel to the sacral nerve plexus, the group of nerves at the base of the spine responsible for bladder function. Because improvement happens gradually, the procedure is performed in a series of half-hour office visits. A second approach stimulates the sacral nerve through a permanently implanted device that resembles a cardiac pacemaker, placed under the skin in the buttock area. Both approaches are moderately successful for alleviating urge incontinence.

**Injections.** Collagen and other bulking agents can be injected around the urethra to create a tighter seal between it and the bladder. The procedure is used primarily for stress incontinence. Urethral injections often need to be repeated. They are usually reserved for people who are unwilling or unable to undergo surgery.

**Surgery.** Several bladder suspension procedures are designed to raise the bladder and urethra with a sling of tissue or a mesh of synthetic material to prevent urine from leaking. At least two sling procedures can be performed through tiny incisions under local anesthetic. However, the FDA has cautioned that inserting surgical mesh slings through vaginal incisions is associated with higher rates of side effects—including severe pelvic pain and organ perforations—than other pelvic floor procedures. Hysterectomy may be done at the same time as bladder suspension procedures when incontinence is accompanied by uterine prolapse (see "Pelvic organ prolapse," page 49).

## Treating fecal incontinence

Although the circumstances of fecal incontinence are somewhat different from those of urinary incontinence, the treatments are similar. They are directed at controlling diarrhea and constipation by adding more fiber to the diet, strengthening the pelvic muscles, and improving the ability of the anal sphincter to contract.

**Pelvic muscle strengthening.** Kegel exercises can strengthen pelvic floor and sphincter muscles. Biofeedback training offers much the same benefit, but in addition to helping you strengthen and coordinate the action of your sphincter muscles, it can improve your ability to sense the presence of stool in the rectum. It offers a 75% chance of improvement and a 50% chance of complete relief.

Electrical and magnetic stimulation of pelvic floor muscles may also be used to treat fecal incontinence, but there are few data on the effectiveness of either.

**Surgery.** If you do require surgery, the exact approach will depend on the cause of your symptoms and your response to previous treatments. The operations include procedures to correct rectal prolapse; to repair and raise the pelvic floor muscles; and to reshape, repair, and replace the anal sphincter. Colostomy is a last resort. This procedure involves bringing the end of the intestine to a surgical opening in the patient's abdomen. Feces are collected in a small pouch worn over the opening.

# Skin cancers

If, like many women, you are finding that the face in the mirror doesn't match the image in your head, skin aging is likely to be responsible. However, the single biggest cause of damage to skin over time is not aging, but sun exposure. Over the years, sun exposure causes fine and coarse wrinkles; baggy skin with a yellow, leathery appearance; and pigmented areas known as lentigines or age spots. And because sun exposure diminishes collagen, which supports a network of blood vessels, photoaging can also cause skin to bruise more easily.

The most serious effect of sun exposure, though, is that it increases the risk for skin cancer. In fact, ultraviolet radiation from the sun is the most important cause of skin cancer, and of the premalignant lesions that are the precursors to many skin cancers.

## Precancer

The FDA has estimated that almost half of all skin cancers begin as a thick, scaly, crusty patch of actinic keratosis (AK). A consequence of sun exposure, AK can cause discomfort and itching, but more important, it can develop into squamous cell carcinoma.

Most treatments remove these crusty patches without scarring, providing both cosmetic benefits and skin cancer protection in the bargain. The most common are prescription creams containing either fluorouracil (5-FU) or imiquimod. The 5-FU cream removes AK patches, but it causes sun sensitivity and, often, considerable discomfort. Imiquimod stimulates the immune system to release cytokines, chemicals that fight cancer cells and viruses. The AK patches become inflamed, crust over, and heal.

Widespread facial patches may warrant deeper treatments. Laser resurfacing vaporizes the epidermis and upper dermis; chemical peels dissolve the outer layers of the skin with an acidic solution; and photodynamic therapy employs light to activate a topical solution of aminolevulinic acid, which then destroys the AK cells. Laser resurfacing and chemical peels can involve local or general anesthesia. Depending on how deeply the skin is penetrated, they may result in considerable swelling.

## Basal cell and squamous cell cancers

The least severe form of skin cancer, basal cell carcinoma is also the most common form, accounting for about 80% of cases. It originates in basal cells located deep in the epidermis. A basal cell carcinoma may first appear as a pearly pimple or bump, a white- or yellow-colored scar, a scaly red patch, or a pimple that won't heal. Basal cell cancer is very slow-growing. Although basal cell carcinoma is caused by sun exposure, sunscreens do not seem to protect against it.

Squamous cell carcinoma arises from flat, scale-like cells in the epidermis and often progresses from AK (see "Precancer," at left). Although squamous cell cancer usually isn't fatal, it can be life-threatening if it spreads to lymph nodes or internal organs. But even then, the cure rate is around 50%. It usually starts as a small, scaly bump and grows slowly until it resembles an ulcer or wart. Only one-fourth of squamous cell carcinomas occur in women.

Options for treating basal and squamous cell cancers are similar; in both cases, the cancer and a margin of healthy tissue around it are surgically removed. Other options for superficial skin cancers include cryosurgery with liquid nitrogen, laser surgery, and treatment with the fluorouracil or imiquimod creams used for treating AK.

## Melanoma: The deadliest skin cancer

About 30,000 women every year develop melanoma, which is responsible for more than 75% of skin cancer deaths. Without treatment, melanoma can spread (metastasize) to the lymph nodes and internal organs. It's a good idea to memorize the signs of moles that may have developed melanoma (see "The ABCDEs of melanoma," page 42).

To treat melanoma, the mole and a margin of healthy tissue are removed. At the same time, the surgeon might do a sentinel node biopsy—removing the lymph node nearest the tumor to see if it contains any cancer cells. If it does, additional lymph nodes will be removed in the same procedure. In addition to surgery, standard treatments for melanoma include chemotherapy, radiation, and biological therapy, which strengthens the immune system against the cancer. New targeted molecular treatments promise to extend survival time for people with metastatic melanoma.

Melanoma 10-year survival rates are 95% or higher if the tumor is less than 1 millimeter thick and has not spread beyond the initial site. As with most other forms of cancer, if the tumor has spread to distant organs, survival is lower.

## Protecting against skin cancers

Sun damage that sets the stage for skin cancer is caused by ultraviolet (UV) radiation, mainly UVA and UVB. For the best protection, choose a sunscreen that has an SPF (sun protection factor) rating of at least 15 and shields against both UVA and UVB. Slather it plentifully on all exposed skin 20 minutes before going out in the sun and every two hours thereafter if you stay outside. If you have fair skin or expect to be in the sun for several hours, a broad-brimmed hat and protective clothing can offer additional protection.

If you're taking certain medications, sun exposure can cause additional damage to your skin. Check the labels of any drugs you're taking to see if they cause photosensitivity. The most common of these include the antibiotic doxycycline, hydrochlorothiazide diuretics, and anti-arrhythmics like amiodarone (Cordarone).

# Vision problems

The first sign of age-related eye changes is presbyopia, deterioration of close-up vision. While most of us get around that with a pair (or several pairs) of drugstore readers or progressive lenses, more serious age-related eye problems can cause vision loss or visual distortion that glasses can't fix. However, newer therapies are reducing vision loss.

## Cataracts

A cataract is a clouding of the normally clear lens of the eye. It is painless and progresses slowly. Vision usually turns blurry, hazy, or dim, and glare from lights and the sun can be distressing. Night vision worsens, and colors appear duller. Cataracts can be easily detected during an eye exam.

Cataracts are primarily due to age-related changes in the lens. However, eating plenty of fruits and vegetables, which contain an abundance of antioxidant vitamins, may lower the risk of developing cataracts. Sunglasses can offer protection against UV radiation, which also contributes to cataracts.

Surgery for cataracts—removing and replacing the clouded lens—is now an outpatient procedure that takes less than an hour. Recovery time is short—often a day or two. These days, there is little reason to put off surgery if cataracts are affecting your quality of life.

## Glaucoma

Many factors may contribute to glaucoma, a condition marked by high pressure inside the eye. If it goes untreated, the excess pressure on the optic nerve slowly erodes vision, beginning with peripheral vision and gradually closing in until central vision goes as well. If glaucoma is detected early, its progression can be halted or slowed, often with prescription eye drops. For more advanced glaucoma, laser treatments or surgery may be necessary.

Because early glaucoma usually causes no symptoms, regular glaucoma screening is recommended for

---

## The ABCDEs of melanoma

If a spot on your skin meets any of the criteria below, be sure to see a dermatologist right away.

**Asymmetry.** Most moles have a round, symmetrical shape, but melanoma is asymmetrical, meaning one side may be different in shape than the other.

**Border irregularity.** Normal moles are round and typically have a clear border. In melanoma, the borders are shabby, uneven, or indistinct, sometimes blending into the surrounding skin. A mole resembling the shape of cauliflower, for instance, should be checked out.

**Color.** Melanomas are usually very dark, but often are a mix of hues rather than one color.

**Diameter.** Most common moles are small, less than 5 millimeters, which is about a quarter of an inch. Melanoma grows, so talk to your doctor if the spot is larger than that.

**Evolving.** Look for any change in size, shape, color, or elevation, or any new symptoms such as bleeding, itching, or crusting.

---

people over 60 and those who have a family history of the disease, are African American or Asian, or are very nearsighted or farsighted. The standard tests for glaucoma involve measuring the pressure inside the eye, doing a test of peripheral vision, and looking for signs of deterioration of the optic nerve.

## Age-related macular degeneration

Among the vision problems that plague older women, age-related macular degeneration (AMD) is perhaps the most serious. As the name implies, macular degeneration is a disease involving the macula, the sensitive central part of the retina (see Figure 8, below). When it begins to deteriorate, central vision worsens.

Nine out of 10 people with AMD have the dry form of this disease, which progresses slowly through early, intermediate, and advanced stages. The remaining 10% have wet AMD, which begins as the dry form and is characterized by the sudden growth of abnor-mal new blood vessels in the layer of cells behind the macula. These new blood vessels are prone to leaking fluid and blood, which damage tissue and photoreceptor cells. The result is scarring and marked loss of vision, usually in the center of the macula. By definition, wet AMD is an advanced form of the disease, and vision loss can occur suddenly.

Smoking increases the risk of developing both types of AMD. Diets low in green, leafy vegetables and high in fat are also associated with AMD. The progression of intermediate dry AMD may be slowed by supplements containing antioxidant vitamins and zinc. When caught early, wet AMD may be slowed with drugs that arrest blood vessel growth or laser treatments.

# Fibromyalgia

Fibromyalgia is a source of frustration to both the women who have it and the clinicians who treat them. If you are one of the more than five million women who live with fibromyalgia, you probably know that it won't kill you and it won't damage your organs and tissues. Yet fibromyalgia can be as disabling as any serious medical condition.

The salient feature of fibromyalgia is a set of "tender points," specific places on the neck, shoulders, arms, back, hips, and legs that hurt when they are pressed (see Figure 9, page 44). Yet most people with fibromyalgia also have a number of other symptoms—generalized muscle pain, fatigue, morning stiffness, headaches, tingling hands and feet, and sleep disturbances. Memory and concentration problems are so common that they've been dubbed "fibro fog." Researchers have yet to identify a cause, although they continue to look for genes, triggering events, and underlying illnesses. One hypothesis is that the condition may be rooted in the central nervous system, resulting in acute sensitivity to pain.

## Treating fibromyalgia

Because no underlying disease process is known, medical treatment is aimed at treating symptoms. It can involve muscle relaxants, medications to relieve pain, and low-dose antidepressants to improve mood,

## Figure 8: The anatomy of the eye

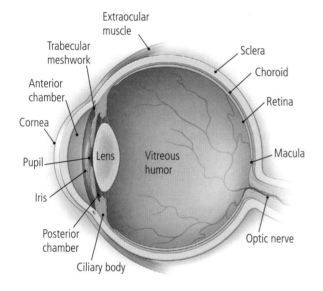

Rays of light pass through the cornea, the anterior chamber, and then through the lens, which focuses images. The lens is nourished by the aqueous humor, a clear, watery solution that circulates from the posterior chamber into the anterior chamber and helps maintain normal pressure. Light reaches the retina after it passes from the lens through the vitreous humor, a clear gel that fills most of the eyeball. The retina has light-sensitive cells that capture images, which are then sent to the brain via the optic nerve. At the retina's center is the macula, a small region that provides sharp, central vision.

## Figure 9: Tender points of fibromyalgia

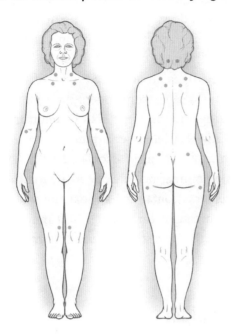

Areas of tissue that become painful when pressed, particularly in the locations shown, are called "tender points." They often develop in people with fibromyalgia, occur less frequently in people with other conditions (such as chronic fatigue syndrome), and are rare in healthy individuals.

fatigue, and sleep. Three drugs have been approved expressly for treating fibromyalgia: pregabalin (Lyrica), an antiseizure medication that blocks pain signals from the central nervous system, and the antidepressants duloxetine (Cymbalta) and milnacipran (Savella).

One of the most effective treatments for fibromyalgia is to take very good care of yourself. A routine of gentle stretching exercises and low-impact aerobic exercise, like swimming or cycling, is very important in relieving stiffness and preserving muscle tone. Adequate sleep, naturally, is also essential to minimizing fatigue. Many women with fibromyalgia have reported benefits from acupuncture and massage therapy as well as from practicing biofeedback, relaxation, and stress reduction. Finally, the value of psychological support can't be underrated when dealing with an often puzzling chronic condition. You may find a fibromyalgia support group in your area through the National Fibromyalgia Association (www.fmaware.org).

# Irritable bowel syndrome

Irritable bowel syndrome (IBS) is medically defined as abdominal pain or discomfort that occurs in association with altered bowel habits over a period of at least three months. If you have IBS, you probably recognize it as recurrent bouts of constipation, diarrhea, or both, as well as abdominal pain, bloating, and gas. IBS hasn't been attributed to an underlying disease process or structural abnormality. It is thought to involve various, often interacting, factors—infection, faulty brain-gut communication, heightened pain sensitivity, hormones, allergies, and emotional stress.

### Treating IBS

Managing IBS is typically a trial-and-error process—first to rule out other conditions, then to find the best way to manage symptoms. According to recommendations from the American College of Gastroenterology (ACG), extensive testing is unnecessary if you have typical IBS symptoms and no family history or symptoms of colon cancer, inflammatory bowel disease, or celiac disease. There's no cure for IBS, but two general approaches—exercise and dietary changes—may reduce the frequency and severity of episodes.

**Exercise.** Many doctors advise people with IBS to get more exercise, and a 2011 randomized controlled clinical trial validated that recommendation. In that study, 75 people, 56 of whom were women, were divided into two groups. Those in one group were told to increase their activity to 30 minutes of moderate to vigorous exercise three to five times a week. The others were instructed to follow their usual habits. All the participants completed standard questionnaires used to evaluate IBS symptoms at the beginning and end of the 12-week study. The average scores of the exercise group dropped 51 points (indicating improvement) while those of the control group fell only 5 points.

**Dietary changes.** In addition to the changes described later in this section (see "Diarrhea" and "Gas and bloating," page 45), some people benefit from a diet that limits foods containing sugar-like molecules known as FODMAPs, short for fermentable oligo-di-monosaccharides and polyols. These substances promote gas formation and are found in a variety of foods, including milk, some fruits and vegetables, wheat, rye, high-fructose corn syrup, and artificial sweeteners. The low-FODMAP approach requires eliminating foods that are high in FODMAPs and reintroducing them one by one to see which ones trigger symptoms. Because a low-FODMAP diet eliminates some foods that are part of healthy diet, it isn't a good idea to try a low-FODMAP diet on your own. Talk to a nutritionist to work out a reasonable plan and to get some recipes for healthy low-FODMAP meals.

## Targeting specific symptoms

Another approach is to target your treatment not to IBS in general, but to your predominant symptoms, which might include any of the following:

**Constipation.** Bulking agents that contain psyllium (ispaghula husk)—for example, Metamucil, Fiberall, Hydrocil, and Konsyl—improve overall symptoms, but the panel that developed the ACG's recommendations found that neither wheat bran nor corn bran is better than a placebo in managing IBS. Lubiprostone (Amitiza) relieves overall symptoms in women with constipation-predominant IBS, but should not be taken by women who are or could become pregnant. In 2012, the FDA approved linaclotide (Linzess), which eases intestinal pain and helps stool move more quickly through the colon. The ACG experts didn't find much evidence for laxatives, but many clinicians think these may be safe and effective when used judiciously. However, laxatives with stimulant properties (such as Dulcolax, Senokot, and Ex-Lax) may cause some cramping.

**Diarrhea.** Fatty foods, coffee, and alcohol can trigger cramps and diarrhea. So can chewing gum or drinking beverages containing sorbitol (a sugar alcohol) or fructose (a component of honey and fruit), which are used as sweeteners in many food products. Loperamide (Imodium) reduces intestinal contractions and fluid secretion in the gut. It helps relieve diarrhea, but not pain. The prescription drug diphenoxylate (Lomotil) may also be useful. Another prescription medication, alosetron (Lotronex), is available for women with severe IBS-associated diarrhea who haven't received adequate relief from life-style approaches and other drugs. However, it has been associated with rare but serious side effects, including colon damage. Two additional drugs received FDA approval for treating IBS-associated diarrhea in 2015—rifaximin (Xifaxan), an antibiotic that stays in the gut and was approved for short-term use, and eluxadoline (Viberzi), an opioid that reduces bowel contractions. However, both have demonstrated only modest improvements over a dummy pill (placebo) in clinical trials.

**Gas and bloating.** The best approach is to try eliminating foods that tend to trigger these symptoms. Common offenders are beans, pretzels, bagels, milk products, carbonated beverages, raw fruits such as bananas and apples, and vegetables such as cabbage, cauliflower, and broccoli. It's also important to rule out celiac disease, gluten sensitivity, or lactose intolerance as a cause of symptoms. Most drugs, either prescription or over the counter, aren't very effective.

**Pain.** A heating pad may ease abdominal pain, and caffeine-free herbal tea such as chamomile can be soothing. Some people have found that peppermint oil helps reduce spasms. However, people who have gastroesophageal reflux disease, or GERD, should avoid peppermint oil, because it can make reflux symptoms worse. Antispasmodics—including dicyclomine (Bentyl) and hyoscyamine (Anaspaz, Cystospaz, Levsin, others)—may help relieve pain by reducing bowel spasms. Low doses of tricyclic antidepressants and SSRIs may alleviate abdominal pain and relieve other symptoms as well.

**Overall symptoms.** Psychological therapies, including cognitive therapy, psychodynamic psychotherapy, and hypnotherapy—but not relaxation therapy—have been found to work better than usual care in relieving overall symptoms. There is some evidence that probiotics may be effective. *Lactobacillus* alone apparently doesn't relieve IBS symptoms, but *Bifidobacterium* and certain combination products may help. Short-term use of rifaximin helps reduce symptoms, especially bloating. However, its long-term safety and effectiveness are uncertain. Moreover, it is very expensive. ▼

# Managing problems unique to women

Most of the topics covered in this Special Health Report affect men as well as women—although sometimes in different ways or in different proportions. But some of the most bothersome health problems that start occurring in middle age are unique to women because they originate in the reproductive system. This chapter discusses noncancerous problems. (For breast cancer and ovarian cancer, see pages 14 and 18, respectively.)

## Persistent menopausal symptoms

Although some women breeze through menopause, others have symptoms that persist for years after their last period. In fact, a 2015 report from the Study of Women's Health Across the Nation (SWAN), a long-term study of women of different races and ethnicities who are in the menopausal transition, indicated that symptoms last on average seven years, but may persist as long as 14 years. Research has helped to identify the approaches that are most effective in relieving symptoms.

### Hormones or not?

The history of hormone therapy has been confusing. But one thing is clear: if you have severe menopausal symptoms, nothing delivers more effective relief than hormone therapy, using a combination of estrogen and progestin. (You must use both unless you've had a hysterectomy; taking estrogen alone raises your risk of endometrial cancer in the uterine lining.) The question isn't how effective hormones are at relieving menopausal symptoms. It's how much risk is entailed.

Major questions were raised about hormones in 2002, when the Women's Health Initiative (WHI), the largest and longest clinical trial of postmenopausal hormone therapy, released its first findings. The researchers made national headlines when they

reported that Prempro (a combination of estrogen and progestin) increased a woman's risk of heart attacks, strokes, deep-vein thrombosis, pulmonary embolisms, and breast cancer. Women jettisoned their hormones en masse.

However, more recent research suggests that hormone use during the first few years of menopause is not as risky as the WHI researchers initially indicated. To understand why, it helps to know a little about

## What about bioidenticals?

Bioidentical hormones—which the Endocrine Society defines as "compounds that have exactly the same chemical and molecular structure as hormones that are produced in the human body"—are increasingly being used as alternatives to synthetic hormones like Premarin (conjugated equine estrogens) and Prempro (conjugated equine estrogens plus medroxyprogesterone acetate). They are often prepared at compounding pharmacies according to a clinician's prescription and touted as "natural" alternatives to "synthetic" brand-name drugs. However, their portrayal in some books and magazines has been highly misleading. Advocates imply that the hormones provided by compounding pharmacies are more precise copies of a woman's hormones than those produced by pharmaceutical companies. This is incorrect. In fact, many of the FDA-approved estrogen products on the market today fit the definition of bioidentical. What's more, they're made from the same ingredients from the identical suppliers as the compounded versions.

Furthermore, despite advertising claims, there is very little medical evidence that bioidenticals are any more beneficial than Premarin and Prempro. And unlike the FDA-approved bioidenticals, those from compounding pharmacies haven't undergone the scrutiny and clinical testing required for approval by the FDA, nor do they come with the same guarantees of dose and purity. In fact, a 2015 survey of postmenopausal women commissioned by the North American Menopause Society indicated that women who used compounded hormones had a higher rate of endometrial cancer, compared with those who relied on pharmaceutical hormones.

the design of the study. The researchers' goal was not to demonstrate relief from menopausal symptoms (which was already well established), but to provide scientific evidence that hormones could also deliver a broader set of presumed benefits, including protection against heart disease, Alzheimer's, and a host of age-related problems. For this reason, they enrolled women in their 50s, 60s, and 70s who had never taken hormones before. This group obviously included many women without menopausal symptoms.

As it turned out, the increased risks, which were slight, were mainly in those who began taking hormones more than 10 years after menopause. By contrast, for those under 60 and within 10 years of menopause, both heart disease and diabetes risk actually went down. (The same was not true of breast cancer. Risk increased in the younger women who were taking a combination of estrogen and progestin.)

What does this mean for women seeking relief from menopausal symptoms? Your decision whether to use hormone therapy largely depends on two things—the severity of your symptoms and whether or not you have what doctors call contraindications, meaning reasons why a particular treatment is not advisable in your case. The latter would include a history of breast, uterine, or endometrial cancer, all of which can be driven by estrogen. Estrogen also increases the risk of seizures, so if you have epilepsy, hormone therapy is not a good bet for you. And anyone with a history of liver problems or unwanted clotting (either during pregnancy or while taking oral contraceptives) should not take estrogen in pill form. That's because the estrogen in oral formulations is processed in the liver, which, in response, increases its production of chemicals that promote clotting—a probable explanation for some of the increased risk of heart attacks and strokes in WHI.

If there are no reasons for you to avoid hormones, you should then consider how troublesome your symptoms are. If you have moderate to severe symptoms—such as debilitating hot flashes and night sweats that continually rob you of sleep—hormone therapy can go a long way toward improving your quality of life. It is also very effective for vaginal dryness. Still, doctors recommend that women use the smallest effective dose of hormones for the shortest possible time needed to obtain relief. For those with vaginal symptoms, low-dose vaginal estrogen may be sufficient (see Table 6, below). It's applied locally, and very little of it gets into the rest of the body. For those with more bothersome symptoms, higher-dose hormones are available in many different forms, including pills, patches, creams, and sprays (see Table 7, page 48).

## Nonhormonal approaches to menopausal symptoms

Understandably, interest in alternatives to hormone therapy has surged. But because nonhormonal treatments don't fully address menopausal complaints, many women concentrate on relieving their most troublesome symptoms first. A combination of lifestyle changes, over-the-counter remedies, and prescription drugs can often provide enough relief to make life tolerable.

The following is a symptom-by-symptom review of some of the most successful nonhormonal approaches.

**Hot flashes.** Dress in layers that are easily shed. A number of websites offer moisture-wicking cloth-

---

### Table 6: Low-dose vaginal estrogen therapy for vaginal atrophy

These products, which contain low doses of estrogen, can reverse tissue thinning, dryness, and other age-related changes of the vagina without significantly increasing blood estrogen levels.

| FORM | TRADE NAME(S) | HOW IT'S USED |
|------|---------------|---------------|
| Cream | Estrace, Ogen, Premarin | Small amount of cream inserted into the vagina on a prescribed schedule |
| Ring | Estring | Small ring inserted into the vagina once every three months |
| Tablet | Vagifem | Small tablet inserted into the vagina nightly for two weeks at the start of treatment and then twice a week |

Note: Although the package inserts for these products currently describe the same risks as for systemic hormonal medications, the risks are in fact much lower, since only minimal amounts of hormones are absorbed into the bloodstream.

## Table 7: Hormone therapy for menopausal symptoms

These products increase blood levels of estrogen and treat both vaginal dryness and other menopausal symptoms such as hot flashes and night sweats. Women without a uterus can take estrogen by itself; those who have a uterus must take a progestin or progesterone in addition to estrogen (either separately or in a combination product) to minimize the risk of uterine cancer that can occur with estrogen alone.

| HORMONE(S) | TRADE NAME |
| --- | --- |
| **Oral estrogen** | |
| conjugated equine estrogens | Premarin |
| synthetic conjugated estrogens | Cenestin, Enjuvia |
| esterified estrogens | Menest |
| 17ß-estradiol* | Estrace, generics |
| estrone (estropipate) | Ogen, Ortho-Est, generics |
| **Transdermal estrogen** | |
| 17ß-estradiol* | Alora, Climara, Esclim, Estraderm, Menostar, Minivelle, Vivelle-Dot, generics (patches); Divigel, Elestrin, Estrogel (gels); Estrasorb (cream); Evamist (spray) |
| **Vaginal estrogen** | |
| estradiol acetate | Femring (ring) |
| **Oral progestin** | |
| medroxyprogesterone acetate | Provera, generics |
| norethindrone | Micronor, Nor-QD, generics |
| megestrol acetate | Megace |
| **Intrauterine progestin** | |
| levonorgestrel | Mirena (intrauterine device) |
| **Oral progesterone** | |
| micronized progesterone | Prometrium |
| **Vaginal progesterone** | |
| progesterone | Crinone 8% (gel); Endometrin (vaginal tablet) |
| **Oral combination estrogen-progestogen** | |
| conjugated estrogens plus medroxyprogesterone acetate | Premphase, Prempro |
| ethinyl estradiol plus norethindrone acetate | Femhrt |
| 17ß-estradiol plus norethindrone acetate* | Activella |
| 17ß-estradiol plus norgestimate* | Prefest |
| **Transdermal combination estrogen-progestogen** | |
| 17ß-estradiol plus norethindrone acetate* | CombiPatch (patch) |
| 17ß-estradiol plus levonorgestrel* | Climara Pro (patch) |

*ß = beta. Source: FDA.

ing for women who have hot flashes. Keep one room in your home cool and retreat to it when flashes start. Try plunging your hands in cold water and then patting your face, neck, and chest. Deep breathing exercises, initiated at the beginning of a hot flash, may nip it in the bud. Or keep a small fan near your workspace or chair.

**Sleep disturbances.** Although it's debatable whether hot flashes are the sole culprit for lost sleep, they are certainly implicated. Sleeping in a cool room and using bedding and nightwear made of materials that wick moisture away from the body may prevent you from waking drenched at 2 a.m.

**Vaginal dryness.** Two types of products—lubricants and moisturizers—can relieve dryness and itching. They can also make sexual intercourse (which in itself can stimulate natural lubrication) more comfortable in women with dyspareunia (pain during intercourse). Lubricants, like Astroglide and K-Y Sensual Silk, are water-based and pH neutral. They approximate the feel of vaginal secretions and provide temporary relief. Moisturizers, like K-Y Liquibeads and Replens, cling to the cells lining the vaginal wall for longer-lasting effectiveness. At least one clinical study has documented that Replens, like estrogen cream, increases the thickness of the vaginal lining.

**Depression.** Prescription antidepressants can do double duty in menopause, relieving both depression and hot flashes. Those shown to work for both conditions in clinical trials include venlafaxine (Effexor), 25 to 150 mg daily; fluoxetine (Prozac), 20 mg daily for four weeks; and paroxetine (Paxil), 10 to 20 mg daily.

**Memory lapses.** The SWAN study has suggested that memory lapses and cognitive problems are temporary, resolving after menopause. In the meantime, it may help to keep detailed to-do lists and take careful notes.

**Overall symptom relief.** Regular exercise can do a world of good. It not only helps keep your body temperature on an even keel, but it can also elevate your mood and help you sleep more soundly. Moreover, it is a memory aid. A study in women ages 50 to 63 indicated that the more the women engaged in moderate exercise, such as brisk walking, the better their memories were.

# Pelvic organ prolapse

As many as one-third of women at midlife have some kind of pelvic organ prolapse—a condition in which uterine, bladder, urethral, or rectal tissue protrudes into the vagina (see Figure 10, below). It is one of the most common causes of incontinence.

The risk of pelvic organ prolapse increases with age, and it's more common in women who've given birth, either by cesarean or vaginally. Other contributing factors may include family history, excess weight, weak connective tissue, chronic constipation, and an occupation that requires heavy lifting.

## Treating pelvic organ prolapse

Some women with pelvic organ prolapse use a pessary, a device similar to a diaphragm that's inserted in the vagina, to help support the pelvic area. Other techniques that may help are Kegel exercises, which involve contracting and relaxing pelvic floor muscles, and physical therapy involving biofeedback or a massage-like technique called myofascial release.

Surgery to repair ligaments supporting pelvic organs and areas of weakened vaginal tissue is an option for women who suffer from symptoms of pelvic organ prolapse. Symptoms may include a bulge or vaginal pressure, along with urinary, defecatory, or sexual dysfunction. In the past, symptoms such as low back or pelvic pain were often been attributed to pelvic organ prolapse, but this association has been disproved.

**Hysterectomy.** For women who have completed childbearing, hysterectomy is an option. This procedure is often combined with ligament and tissue repair as well as procedures to address any associated incontinence (see "Treating urinary incontinence," page 39). Because the tissues involved can lose elasticity over the years, some women may need surgery redone after some time.

Although almost one-third of women have had a hysterectomy by age 60, less than 20% of the procedures are performed in women 55 or older. That's because two of the most common conditions associated with hysterectomy—fibroids and endometriosis—usually regress after menopause. In older women, most hysterectomies are performed for one of two reasons: pelvic floor prolapse or cancer (including precancerous conditions). Other common reasons for hysterectomy are bleeding and pain. Hysterectomy has become less common as alternative treatment options have developed.

Hysterectomy can be done laparoscopically (using scopes and surgical instruments inserted through small incisions in the vagina or abdomen), either manually or robot-assisted, and is often performed by combining these methods, such as in laparoscopically assisted vaginal hysterectomy or laparoscopic hysterectomy using a small abdominal incision to remove the uterus. The "Band-Aid" incisions involved in laparoscopic approaches allow for a quick recovery.

The type of procedure depends upon the reason for the hysterectomy, your anatomy and medical issues, and a balancing of risks and personal preferences. Abdominal procedures (with or without laparoscopy) are usually necessary when a hysterectomy is performed to treat cancer. Vaginal surgery, which leaves no visible scar and has a shorter recovery period, is a good option for uterine prolapse and other benign conditions. Whether it is appropriate often depends on the size of the uterus; fibroids can make the organ too bulky to remove through a vaginal incision.

## Figure 10: Normal positions of the pelvic organs

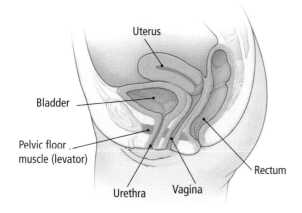

In pelvic organ prolapse, the pelvic floor muscles that support the organs are weakened. One or more of the organs shift from their normal positions and can press against the walls of the vagina.

## Figure 11: Types of hysterectomy

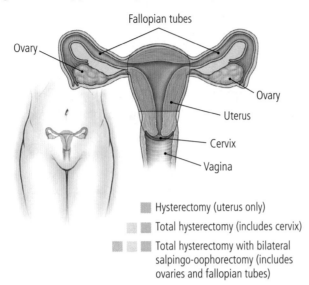

Hysterectomy (uterus only)

Total hysterectomy (includes cervix)

Total hysterectomy with bilateral salpingo-oophorectomy (includes ovaries and fallopian tubes)

In older women, most hysterectomies are usually performed for one of two reasons—pelvic floor prolapse or cancer, including precancerous conditions. The ovaries may be removed along with the uterus in order to prevent or treat ovarian cancer, but this will interrupt the production of small amounts of testosterone and DHEA, which continues after menopause.

Should you also remove the ovaries (and fallopian tubes)? The ovaries were once routinely removed when postmenopausal women were having a hysterectomy (see Figure 11, above), and they still are when the rea-son is cancer. The decision seems reasonable: removing the tubes and ovaries reduces (but does not eliminate) the risk of ovarian cancer. However, the postmeno-pausal ovary is not totally inactive after menopause; while estrogen production stops, small amounts of the hormones testosterone and DHEA continue to be pro-duced into the eighth decade of life.

A growing body of evidence suggests that surgi-cal removal of the ovaries at the time of hysterectomy may have long-term health consequences, and the risks are greater for women who are younger at the time of removal and have not used estrogen therapy. Data from the Nurses' Health Study and other studies indicate that when a woman has a hysterectomy for a benign condition, her risk of breast or ovarian cancer declines, but her likelihood of developing heart dis-ease, stroke, and lung cancer goes up. In fact, losing her ovaries increases her risk of dying from any cause. Some women, as a compromise, are having the fallo-pian tubes removed but not the ovaries; this appears to reduce the risk of ovarian cancer, but not to the same extent as removal of both the tubes and ovaries. Stay tuned for more studies on this.

If you're considering a hysterectomy for pelvic prolapse or any other benign condition, discuss the risks and benefits of conserving your ovaries with your doctor. ▼

# Embracing the future

Aging is more a winding path than a downhill slalom. Changes in brain function as well as your outlook on life can influence the journey ahead.

## Your aging brain—the upsides

If you forget a name or two, take longer to finish the crossword, or find it hard to manage two tasks at once, don't assume you're on the road to dementia. What you're experiencing is age-related changes in the way your brain works. And in many ways it's actually working better. Studies have shown that older people have better judgment, are better at making rational decisions, and are better able to screen out negativity than their juniors.

The brain compensates for a slower processing speed by using more of itself. MRIs taken of a teenager working through a problem show a lot of activity on one side of the prefrontal cortex, the region we use for conscious reasoning. In middle age, the other side of the brain begins to pitch in a little. In seniors, both sides of the brain are sharing the task equally. A host of studies in the last decade have shown that the more mature brain actually has advantages over its younger counterpart. For example, in a study of air traffic controllers and airline pilots, those between ages 50 and 69 took longer than those under 50 to master new equipment, but once they had, they made fewer mistakes using it. (Keep this in mind when you're trying to conquer a new computer program or adapt to a new car!)

At midlife you are probably better at the following:

- **Inductive reasoning.** Older people are less likely to rush to judgment and more likely to reach the right conclusion based on the information. This is an enormous help in everyday problem solving, from planning the most efficient way to do your errands to figuring out why the hot water isn't flowing in the kitchen sink.

- **Verbal abilities.** In middle age, you continue to expand your vocabulary and hone your ability to express yourself.
- **Spatial reasoning.** Remember those quizzes that required you to identify an object that had been turned around? You are likely to score better on them in your 50s and 60s than you did in your teens. And you may be a better driver, too.
- **Basic math.** You may be better at splitting the check and figuring the tip when you're lunching with friends, simply because you've been doing it for so many years.

## Your outlook on aging—and how it can help you

"Age is only a number" and "You're as young as you feel" are more than platitudes. A growing body of research has indicated that attitudes toward aging have a strong effect on health and longevity. People who have a positive view of aging are less likely to develop cardiovascular disease, dementia, and other chronic conditions. And a recent study of 6,500 seniors indicated that those who reported feeling at least three years younger than their calendar age had a significantly lower death rate over the next eight years compared with those who felt their age or older.

One of the most encouraging reports on the relationship of attitudes and longevity was published by Yale psychologist Becca Levy and colleagues in 2002. That team had analyzed data in the Ohio Longitudinal Study of Aging and Retirement—a project that followed more than 1,000 residents of Oxford, Ohio, who were over 50 in 1975. All participants were asked about their views on aging and older people at the beginning of the study. Researchers followed the participants for 23 years, noting who developed chronic illnesses and who died. They found that the men and women who had expressed a sanguine attitude toward old age tended to live 7.5 years longer than those who had a dimmer view of aging. More recent research has linked negative attitudes about aging to an increased risk of cardiovascular disease, dementia, and even the brain changes that precede dementia.

## How to achieve a positive attitude

Over the last decade, researchers have identified practices that can help you achieve and sustain a positive attitude toward your future. Many of them are explained in the Harvard Special Health Report *Positive Psychology* (see "Resources," page 53). Here are a few quick suggestions:

**Savor pleasure.** Savoring pleasure is placing your attention on something pleasing as it occurs, consciously enjoying the experience as it unfolds. Most people are primed to experience pleasure in special moments, such as a wedding day or a vacation. Everyday pleasures, on the other hand, can slip by without much notice unless they disappear or seem threatened. Slow down and focus. You will enjoy things more, whether a meal or a visit with a friend.

**Practice gratitude.** Gratitude is a thankful appreciation for what you receive, whether tangible or intangible. Try keeping a gratitude journal, in which you regularly write down things for which you are grateful. Doing so will help you go through your days with greater appreciation, taking fewer blessings for granted. As you write, be specific and try to relive the sensations you felt as you remember what each thing means to you.

**Cultivate mindfulness.** Mindfulness is generally acquired by training the mind to focus its attention on the present moment in a systematic way, accepting whatever arises. While savoring involves appreciating pleasurable sensations, mindfulness involves opening fully to both pleasant and unpleasant experiences. Being mindful helps you become fully engaged in activities and creates a greater capacity to deal with adverse events. By focusing on the here and now, many people who practice mindfulness find that they are less likely to get caught up in worries about the future or regrets over the past, are less preoccupied with concerns about success and self-esteem, and are better able to form deep connections with others.

**Retain a sense of purpose.** It's normal to experience a sense of loss and even grief when your children leave home, you retire, or you lose a loved one. It's important at these times to maintain as much normalcy in your life as possible, with a regular sleep schedule, exercise, good diet, and social interactions. In many cases, you can view this important life change, no matter how painful, as a new challenge or opportunity. Focus on what's possible. Perhaps you can organize a family reunion or plunge into a volunteer activity you haven't had time for. Doing so should open new horizons.

**Emphasize the positive.** Older people are better than younger people at winnowing out and focusing on the positive aspects of a situation. Doing so is a key factor in acquiring resilience—the ability to bounce back from bad times—that will help you weather the losses that may occur in the years ahead.

You may even find that adopting a positive attitude comes naturally with age. Studies have shown that people over 60 tend to brood less, perhaps because the amygdala, the area of the brain that consolidates emotion and memory, is less responsive to negatively charged situations.

Finally, on survey after survey, older people report that they have become more satisfied with their lives as they have aged, despite the losses that accumulate with passing years. This is most likely because they tend to minimize the negative, accept their limitations and use their experience to compensate for them, and set reasonable goals for the future. ◆